PSYCHIATRY - THEORY, APPLICATIONS, AND TREATMENTS

PSYCHIATRIC RESEARCH TRENDS: DREAMS AND GERIATRIC PSYCHIATRY

PSYCHIATRY - THEORY, APPLICATIONS, AND TREATMENTS

Attention Deficit Hyperactivity Disorder (ADHD)
Stuart M. Gordon and Aileen E. Mitchell (Editors)
2009. ISBN: 978-1-60741-581-7
2009. ISBN: 978-1-60876-699-4 (E-book)

Victimhood, Vengefulness, and the Culture of Forgiveness
Ivan Urlić, Miriam Berger and Avi Berman
2010. ISBN: 978-1-60876-191-3

Psychiatric Research Trends: Dreams and Geriatric Psychiatry
Daniella M. Montez (Editor)
2010. ISBN: 978-1-60741-760-6
2010. ISBN: 978-1-61668-719-9 (E-book)

Optimization of Research and Clinical Applications for Combat-related Posttraumatic Stress Disorder (PTSD): Progress Through Modern Translational Methodologies
Seth D. Norrholm, Tanja Jovanovic, Barbara O. Rothbaum, Michael Davis, Wendy Hasenkamp, Chris Crowe, Erica Duncan, Linda Leimbach, Kelly Skelton and Bekh Bradley
2010. ISBN: 978-1-61668-027-5
2010. ISBN: 978-1-61668-358-0 (E-book)

War and Suicide
Leo Sher and Alexander Vilens (Editors)
2010. ISBN: 978-1-60741-978-5
2010. ISBN: 978-1-61668-274-3 (E-book)

Post-Traumatic Stress Disorder (PTSD): Causes, Symptoms and Treatment
Sylvia J. Egan (Editor)
2010. ISBN: 978-1-61668-526-3
2010. ISBN: 978-1-61668-716-8 (E-book)

Dyslexia and Depression: The Hidden Sorrow
Neil Alexander-Passe
2010. ISBN: 978-1-60876-118-0
2010. ISBN: 978-1-61668-933-9 (E-book)

Stress of Family Members in Caring for a Relative with Schizophrenia
Wai-Tong Chien
2010. ISBN: 978-1-60876-145-6

Military Psychiatry: New Developments
Dennis G. Stanton and Lawrence R. Castaneda (Editors)
2010. ISBN: 978-1-60876-149-4

"Paranoia of the Millionaire": Harry K. Thaw's 1907 Insanity Defense
Emil R. Pinta
2010. ISBN: 978-1-60876-988-9

Psychoanalytic Psychotherapy: A Modern Kleinian Approach
Robert Waska
2010. ISBN: 978-1-60876-909-4

Suicidal Behavior in Alcohol and Drug Abuse and Dependence
Leo Sher and Alexander Vilens (Editors)
2010. ISBN: 978-1-60876-919-3

Neurobiology of Post-Traumatic Stress Disorder
Leo Sher and Alexander Vilens (Editors)
2010. ISBN: 978-1-61668-851-6
2010. ISBN: 978-1-61668-816-5 (E-book)

Young, Violent, and Dangerous to Know
Michael Fitzgerald
2010. ISBN: 978-1-60876-952-0

Delusional Misidentification
Garry Young
2010. ISBN: 978-1-60876-956-8

Paranoia in the "Normal" Population
Antonio Preti and Matteo Cella
2010. ISBN: 978-1-60876-984-1

Malingering Versus Posttraumatic Stress Disorder
Kenneth R. Morel
2010. ISBN: 978-1-61668-144-9
2010. ISBN: 978-1-61668-454-9 (E-book)

Cognitive Impairment in Children with ADHD
Alasdair Vance, Catherine Mollica and Paul Maruff
2010. ISBN: 978-1-61668-197-5
2010. ISBN: 978-1-61668-476-1 (E-book)

Immigration and Mental Health: Stress, Psychiatric Disorders and Suicidal Behavior Among Immigrants and Refugees
Leo Sher and Alexander Vilens (Editors)
2010. ISBN: 978-1-61668-503-4

Post-Traumatic Stress Disorder in Refugee Communities: The Importance of Culturally Sensitive Screening, Diagnosis, and Treatment
Theodore W. McDonald and Jaime N. Sand
2010. ISBN: 978-1-61668-7465
2010. ISBN: 978-1-61668-716-8 (E-book)

Police Suicide: Proactive Leadership and Crisis Management Strategies
Thomas E. Baker
2010. ISBN: 978-1-61668-968-1
2010. ISBN: 978-1-61728-650-6 (E-book)

PSYCHIATRY - THEORY, APPLICATIONS, AND TREATMENTS

PSYCHIATRIC RESEARCH TRENDS: DREAMS AND GERIATRIC PSYCHIATRY

DANIELLA M. MONTEZ
EDITOR

Nova Science Publishers, Inc.
New York

For permission to use material from this book please contact us:
Telephone 631-231-7269; Fax 631-231-8175
Web Site: http://www.novapublishers.com

LIBRARY OF CONGRESS CATALOGING-IN-PUBLICATION DATA

Psychiatric research trends : dreams and geriatric psychiatry / editor,
Daniella M. Montez.
p. ; cm.
Includes bibliographical references and index.
ISBN 978-1-60741-760-6 (hardcover)
1. Geriatric psychiatry. 2. Dreams. I. Montez, Daniella M.
[DNLM: 1. Aged. 2. Mental Disorders. 3. Dreams. WT 150 P9668 2010]
RC451.4.A5P755 2010
618.97'689--dc22

2010007619

Published by Nova Science Publishers, Inc. ✦ New York

CONTENTS

PREFACE

Dreams are a series of images, ideas, emotions, and sensations occurring involuntarily in the mind during certain stages of sleep. The content and purpose of dreams are not fully understood, though they have been a topic of speculation and interest throughout recorded history. Dreams and sleep disorders are commonly found among the geriatric population. Several factors may contribute to these sleep disturbances, such as health problems or changes in ones circadian rhythm. This new book gathers the latest research from around the globe in both these fields of study and focuses on such topics as lucid dreaming, dreaming during anesthesia, elderly suicides and depression in the elderly.

Chapter 1 - Depressive illness results in considerable functional disability and decreased quality of life. The prevalence of depression in older persons ranges from 5 to 30%. Older people often have depression concurrent with other illnesses, e.g., cardiovascular disease. Depression can also impact adversely on these disorders.

Current management of depression commonly involves drugs and psychotherapies, which whilst effective, have variable adherance rates. Non-pharmacological therapies offer potentially safer alternative management of depression in older people. Of the psychotherapies, cognitive behaviour therapy and reminiscence and life review have the best supporting evidence for older people. Few lifestyle change modalities have been sufficiently tested to recommend their use with older people. An exception is physical activity. Both endurance and resistance type physical activity has anti-depressant effects for older people with depression.

Older depressed people have much to gain from being physically active. Physical activity offers a therapy where negative events are minimal and benefits can accrue for both physical and mental health status. Physical activity may assist both in the prevention and management of depression in older people. As a health promotion intervention, it has the potential to reduce the risk of depression and to ameliorate co-morbid conditions. Using physical activity as an antidepressant can reduce the need for pharmacological intervention, minimizing iatrogenic and polypharmacy risk that is particularly prevalent for older people.

Chapter 2 - The burden or stress of the informal carer of dependent elderly people is nowadays one of the main mental health problems, mainly due to the increasing number of elderly people in need of care and help from others in the developed countries. The informal caregiver burden affects especially middle-aged women, who are the typical profile of the person in charge of old dependent adults. These women are affected mainly by depression, anxiety and high stress level and of course use a higher number of psychotropic medicines.

Negative impact on physical health also exists such as negative evaluations of their own health, psychosomatic and immunological disorders, cardiovascular problems, and dependency in order to perform the activities of daily life. The caregiver burden, the emotional discomfort, and indicators of the poor state of health also appear as major predictors of the premature institutionalization and mistreatment of the care recipient.

The results of the research, guided in the majority of cases by the theoretical framework of Pearlin by means of his Stress Process Model (Pearlin et al., 1989, 1990; Pearlin, 1991) has determined the choice for the study of the determining variables of the informal caregiver burden. In this sense, scientific thought shows the existence of multiple variables associated with the caregiver burden, among which it is possible to highlight, in Pearlin's terms, that the variables of the care context as well as the primary stress factors comprise a primary generator core of the burden, whereas the secondary stress factors represent the proliferation of the emotional discomfort and burden in other areas of life.

The authors' research has indicated that the psycho-educational intervention programs framed within the respite services jointly with the knowledge of the determining variables of the burden can comprise the best optimal approach in order to effectively deal with the burden problem of the informal caregivers of dependent senior citizens. Regarding this, this chapter reviews the main theories and results of the existing research to date about the concept of the informal caregiver's burden. The explanation of the burden concept, the theoretical approaches which attempt to explain it, the variables which have emerged in the investigation, the predictors of its appearance, as well as the intervention programs developed to relieve the burden, in order to allow us to approach the appropriate solutions to deal with the current social and political reality of this problem.

Chapter 3 - *Introduction:* Delirium is a neuropsychiatric syndrome defined by acute onset, fluctuating course and disturbances of consciousness, attention, orientation, memory, thought, perception and behavior. The course of delirium has often been described as transient, in which recovery is likely to be complete if the underlying etiological factor is cured. Older people, who have delirium, experience a range of poor clinical outcomes including significant increases in cognitive impairment, functional disability, increased length of hospital stay, psychological distress, high rates of institutionalization, and high rates of death, independent of many socio-demographic and clinical variables.

Methods: Databases were searched with the keywords 'delirium' or 'acute confusion' and 'outcome'. The keywords 'cognitive impairment,' 'functional disability', 'length of hospital stay', 'mortality', 'institutionalization', 'psychological stress' have also been used in combination with the former. Studies have been categorized in relation to six outcomes: a) mortality, b) cognitive impairment, c) functional decline, d) length of hospital stay, e) discharge destination, and f) psychological morbidity.

Results: There are methodological problems and heterogeneity in the examined studies. Regarding cognitive impairment the examined studies suggest that delirium is associated with an increased risk of subsequent cognitive decline. Not all studies have found an association of delirium with subsequent functional impairment. Similarly there are conflicting results among studies which examined length of stay. Most studies agree that there is a relationship between delirium and mortality and especially for those with pre-existing dementia. A majority of studies have found that delirium is associated with a high rate of institutional care. A small number of studies have examined the psychological stress that delirium cause patients and also relatives and nurses.

Discussion: Studies generally agree that there is an association of delirium and subsequent cognitive decline and institutionalization. There is no conclusive evidence about the relationship between delirium and functional disability, length of stay or mortality. Given that there is an association between functional decline and cognitive decline, delirium may induce a long term or even permanent cognitive decline which then manifests as functional decline. The contribution of delirium to mortality is complex. Perhaps underling pathophysiological mechanisms common to both delirium and dementia are related to mortality. It is not yet certain that delirium prolongs hospital stay once other confounding factors are controlled for. The notion of subsyndromal delirium is briefly discussed.

Conclusions: There are many methodological and ethical concerns which obstruct delirium research. It is clear from this review that delirium has very serious adverse outcomes and it is necessary to develop biological markers which can allow a focus of preventative measures on those at most risk of developing it.

Chapter 4 - Anxiety as a separate disorder was introduced into the DSM manuals only in 1980, but is now widely recognized as a common mood disorder in the elderly, and in fact its prevalence, reported to range between 10% to 20% may actually be greater than for depressive illness. On the other hand, its assessment and diagnosis is problematic, and therefore, frequently often under-recognized. Conversely, though the elderly may not actually meet the full requirements for anxiety disorder, they still experience enough symptoms which can disrupt their daily lives. The problem is complicated by the fact that elderly persons have a high incidence of somatic symptoms accompanying their physical illnesses, and also that anxiety in the elderly presents with somatic complaints, then their complaints may be interpreted as being part of some physical illness rather than actually been related to their anxiety, somewhat similar to the problem in diagnosing depression in the elderly. Similarly to depression, several screening instruments were developed and validated for the detection of anxiety, but rarely specifically for the elderly. This chapter will describe and define late-life anxiety, the means of diagnosing the disorder relating especially to the difficulties in the elderly, and finally its interaction with depression.

Chapter 5 - Cognitive decline has become a major burden to society, so if one could delay the decline by initiating treatment as early as possible, the savings for both the individual and society would be significant. The importance of relating to Mild Cognitive Impairment concerns the high annual conversion rates of up to 30% for this disorder. Thus, the importance of finding the predictors for further cognitive decline is of the highest priority. Researchers have proposed the use of neuroimaging, biomarkers, use of EEG brain wave patterns, neuropsychological testing or a combination of them. Amongst the neuropsychological clinical entities examined have been the mood disorders depression and anxiety. Depression has been reported to be a predictor for future cognitive decline, but with regard to anxiety, the question is debatable. In some studies of elderly with memory problems, the presence of anxiety was highly predictive of future cognitive decline. However in studies with MCI cohorts, though anxiety is found in up to 40% of MCI sufferers, it was found not to be a predictor. A possible theoretical explanation is that elderly turning for an assessment are at Braak's stage I/II and in those diagnosed with MCI, are at Braak's stage III/IV. At the earlier stages (stage I/II), flow of information via the entorhinal cortex to the hippocampus is impaired resulting in hyperactivity of the alternate pathway of the amygdala, which explains the high prevalence of anxiety. However, by the time a person turns to a specialized cognitive clinic and is diagnosed with amnestic-MCI (stage III /IV) flow via the alternative pathway of the amygdala though present, is now partially impaired. After conversion to dementia (stage V), only a few were still with anxiety since now the pathway to the amygdala was also impaired. In conclusion, anxiety is prominent in persons with amnestic MCI, but this did not predict future cognitive decline, perhaps since persons with MCI turning for cognitive assessment, probably have early onset of dementia. There does however seem to be a trend that those with anxiety and MCI do tend to develop cognitive decline at slight higher rates.

Chapter 6 – For the first time, neurobiology is in the position to confirm one of the main assertions of psychoanalytic theory, i.e. the existence of unconscious phenomena during waking, namely the repression of unwanted memories which are prevented from accessing consciousness. These results confirm and underscore Freud's old description of the bursting-out of unconscious phenomena as evidenced by parapraxes. The censorship responsible for these repression processes is more obvious during waking than during dreaming, in REM sleep. Indeed, the forebrain, which is responsible for mentation, is so disturbed during this sleep stage that it is difficult to find objective criteria of advanced cognitive processes that could support a hypothetical dream-work generated by a censorship process (Gottesmann, 2006b).

Chapter 7 - The elderly population size is increasing due to prolonged life expectancy and falling birth rates worldwide (Shah and McKenzie, 2007). Traditionally, suicide rates increased with ageing. A recent cross-national study of 62 developing and developed countries reported an increase in suicide rates with ageing in males and females in 25 and 27 countries respectively (Shah, 2007a). Thus, suicides in the elderly are an important public health concern. Comprehensive understanding of the substantial worldwide variation in population patterns of suicide may be critical for developing prevention programmes (Knox et al., 2004). While much is known about individual level risk factors (e.g. Conwell et al., 1991; Catell and Jolley, 1995; Harwood et al., 2001), this strategy has limitations in unmasking more distal causes of suicide (Rehkopf and Buka, 2006). Moreover, detailed knowledge of distal causes may have greater public health relevance for universal prevention strategies (Knox et al., 2004).

Ecological studies, either using cross-national or cross-regional correlations or within-country time series analysis, allow examination of the relationship between regional or national aggregate data on elderly suicide rates and regional or national aggregate data on a range of parameters (e.g. socio-economic status) as potential risk or protective factors, and have major implications for public health. The findings of recent studies examining the relationship between elderly suicides and life expectancy, socio-economic status, income inequality, intelligence and educational attainment, fertility rates, urbanisation, societal crime, unemployment rates, gender inequality, population size, growth and dependency ratios, mental health service funding and provision and degree of human development are described.

Chapter 8 - Excluding awareness, which is the post-anesthesia recall of real events, dreaming during anesthesia can be defined as any recalled experience that occurred between induction of general anesthesia and the first return of consciousness after anesthesia. It is a common phenomenon (5-50%) that varies in incidence with the timing of the post-anesthesia interview. Dreaming is most frequently reported by women who are young, healthy, have home dream recall after sleep, receive short propofol-based anesthesia and who emerge from anesthesia rapidly.

Most dreams are short and neutral or pleasant in content, the latter being related to work, family and recreational activities. Rarely, the dream content suggests a 'near-miss' awareness experience that resulted from an inadequate depth of anesthesia and transient return of consciousness, but most dreams appear to occur during a sleep state in the period just before initial arousal from unconsciousness at the end of anesthesia.

This chapter reviews the incidence of dreaming, factors influencing dreaming, the nature and content of dreams and their psychological impact, the timing of dreaming and the evidence as to whether it occurs during or after anesthesia. To date, research about dreaming during anesthesia has largely involved observational clinical studies, but future neurophysiological research should provide more detailed understanding of what appears to be a common, not unpleasant and harmless event.

Chapter 9 - The future of dreams and dreaming as a topic of study is promising. There is a tremendous need to develop educational opportunities that will reach a large portion of the population. Developing training for clinicians to work with dreams in the treatment setting is another area of particular need. It will be a tremendous challenge to expand educational opportunities in all areas of this field. With that said, it is important that educational opportunities be expanded and maintained as a means of supporting the field of dream studies well into the future.

Chapter 10 - Dreams can be considered as a kind of simulation of the real world on a higher cognitive level (Erlacher & Schredl, 2008b). In a dream the dreamer experiences himself as a dream ego within a dream environment. The dream ego can either actively take part in the plot or observe the ongoing dream. The content of dreams can be very diverse regarding a variety of characteristics, ranging from bizarre to realistic, negative to positive emotions, emotional to rational elements, and so on (cf. Schredl & Wittmann, 2005). After awaking from a dream people often state that they perceived their experience within the dream in a similar way as they might have during wakefulness (Schredl & Hofmann, 2003). A simple explanation for the fact that dreams often seem to mimic the real world so perfectly is that the neural processes of the brain which underlie the dream simulation are the same processes that occur during wakefulness (Schredl, 2000). This notion is underlined by the fact that during REM sleep – the sleep state during which most vivid dreaming occurs – the EEG recording shows high activity of the brain in contrast to NREM sleep (Hobson, Pace-Schott, & Stickgold, 2000). Research applying modern imaging tools (PET, fMRI) shows that the dreaming brain reveals for specific brain areas activations similar to wakefulness whereas other areas tend to be inactive (Dang-Vu et al., 2005). Additionally, the specific activation of the brain corresponds to the specific characteristic of the dream experience, e.g. high activity in the visual association cortex causes visual hallucinosis during dreaming (Hobson et al., 2000). In this paper, therefore, I will assume that especially during REM sleep the brain produces a perfect simulation of the real world on a higher cognitive level.

A special kind of nocturnal dreams is lucid dreaming. In a lucid dream the dreamer realizes the dream state and he or she is often able to control the dream simulation and do whatever he or she wants to do. Because the phenomenon of lucid dreaming seems to be hard to grasp, the first part of the paper will focus on several basic aspects of lucid dreaming. The dreaming brain seems to be an excellent choice to study the relationship between the subjective level and the physiological level. In the second part of the paper psychophysiological studies on lucid dreaming will be reviewed. Those studies do support my assumption that the dreaming brain indeed reflects a simulated world on a higher level. In the third part of the paper different applications of lucid dreaming will be discussed. As a final point, some further future directions for lucid dream research will be presented.

In: Psychiatric Research Trends: Dreams and Geriatric Psychiatry ISBN 978-1-60741-760-6
Editors: Daniella M. Montez, pp.1-25

Chapter 1

MANAGEMENT OF DEPRESSION IN OLDER PEOPLE: A ROLE FOR PHYSICAL ACTIVITY

Jane Sims[1], Daniel O'Connor [2] and Colette Browning[1]
[1]Healthy Ageing Research Unit, School of Primary Health Care and Monash Institute of Health Services Research, Monash University,Victoria, Australia
[2] Department of Psychological Medicine, Monash University, Victoria, Australia

ABSTRACT

Depressive illness results in considerable functional disability and decreased quality of life. The prevalence of depression in older persons ranges from 5 to 30%. Older people often have depression concurrent with other illnesses, e.g., cardiovascular disease. Depression can also impact adversely on these disorders.

Current management of depression commonly involves drugs and psychotherapies, which whilst effective, have variable adherance rates. Non-pharmacological therapies offer potentially safer alternative management of depression in older people. Of the psychotherapies, cognitive behaviour therapy and reminiscence and life review have the best supporting evidence for older people. Few lifestyle change modalities have been sufficiently tested to recommend their use with older people. An exception is physical activity. Both endurance and resistance type physical activity has anti-depressant effects for older people with depression.

Older depressed people have much to gain from being physically active. Physical activity offers a therapy where negative events are minimal and benefits can accrue for both physical and mental health status. Physical activity may assist both in the prevention and management of depression in older people. As a health promotion intervention, it has the potential to reduce the risk of depression and to ameliorate co-morbid conditions. Using physical activity as an antidepressant can reduce the need for pharmacological intervention, minimizing iatrogenic and polypharmacy risk that is particularly prevalent for older people.

INTRODUCTION

Depression is a major contributor to the chronic burden of disease in a population and a leading cause of loss of disability adjusted-life-years (Snow et al., 2000). As populations age, depression is set to become the main cause of global disability. By 2020, it is expected that depression will be the second most common cause of disability worldwide. Depression poses a significant economic burden at a societal level, being associated with increased rates of hospitalization and emergency service use.

Amongst mental health problems, depression ranks as a high prevalence condition and warrants particular attention using primary, secondary and tertiary prevention measures. There is a growing evidence base about the range of preventive and therapeutic interventions to manage depression. This chapter will discuss measures suitable for older people with depression. Older people often have depression concurrent with other illnesses, such as cardiovascular disease. Depression can impact adversely on these disorders and their prognosis. Having depression can also impact on a person's family life and relationships, influencing the person's overall health status and quality of life.

The reasons for depression in older people will be briefly discussed. The management of depression within the context of co- morbidities will also be considered. Both pharmacological and non-pharmacological therapies will be explored, focusing on the role of lifestyle interventions, namely physical activity and nutrition. We acknowledge the heterogeneity of the older population: interventions suitable for both community-dwelling and institutionalised older people will be highlighted. We will argue that, given the promising effects of physical activity in the prevention and treatment of depression and its far-reaching benefits for overall health, that physical activity be promoted as a key lifestyle behaviour amongst older people.

PREVALENCE

Depressive symptomatology is common amongst older people. Estimates of the actual prevalence of depression among older people living in the community vary widely, from 10% to 35% (Beekman et al., 2002, Baldwin et al., 2002b, Beekman et al., 1999, Sayer et al., 2000, Regier et al., 1988). The prevalence of major depression and dysthmia tends to decline with age in population surveys. Some researchers have posited that the reduced depression prevalence amongst older people reflects greater emotional stability, a honing of coping skills, reduced daily hassles and resilience (Henderson, 1994). An alternative explanation relates to sampling methodology. Most national surveys and many gerontological surveys exclude those living in institutions such as aged care facilities and long stay hospitals and those with cognitive impairment (O'Connor, 2006). As will be discussed below, prevalence rates are higher in these groups. Prevalence amongst older people is therefore likely to be underestimated due to this sampling and case ascertainment bias. A third explanation is that older people are more likely to attribute depressive symptoms to physical illness (Hasin, 1988), making their responses to generic mental health scales less likely to produce a positive diagnostic classification.

SYMPTOMATOLOGY

The presenting symptoms of depression may be different from those in younger adults, making it difficult to detect. The symptoms may be associated with the person's current social circumstances or their physical health status. Indeed, in older people the symptoms may be masked by physical ill health problems. For example, chronic osteoarthritis or respiratory disease can cause fatigue. Cognitive impairment can cause memory and concentration difficulties. Worrying, irritability and agitation may be commoner than low mood in older people (Sable et al., 2002). Some depressive symptoms may be side effects of medication the older person is taking. The interactive effects of psychological and physical health need to be carefully considered. Psychological distress may be due to physical ill health, such as pain. In turn, unresolved depression or anxiety can exacerbate pain. The somatic and psychological symptoms of depression and anxiety can make diagnosis more difficult (Barraclough, 1997).

There remains a societal perspective that feeling down, tired and socially withdrawn is normal amongst older people. This can mean that older people do not present to their doctor with depressive symptoms. The health professional needs to be proactive in assessing older patients for depression so that it is treated appropriately. There have been several public health campaigns to raise awareness and physicians are receiving enhanced training to assist in the detection of depression. Although older age can be a risk factor for depression, the evidence base shows that age itself is *not* a risk factor, once age-associated factors are accounted for.

We need to be aware of the difference between 'normal' distress and psychological disturbance. Older people unhappy with their current situation may speak about wanting to be dead. This expression may capture their perceived burden on others, or a feeling of apathy.

Depression is often associated with suicidal thoughts (Pearson and Brown, 2000). Since suicidal comments may indicate depression, referral for assessment is necessary. Fortunately in recent years, suicide rates among older aged males have continued to decline: for example, in Australia (by 17% since 1997), the United States (by 9%), and in New Zealand (24%). Whilst most countries and regions have reported decreasing trends of suicide mortality amongst those 65 years or older since the early 1990s (Australian Institute for Suicide Research and Prevention, 2003), there remains an increased risk of completed suicides among older people, especially older men. As many as 90% of individuals who complete suicide have at least one diagnosable mental illness, usually depression. Detection and treatment of mental illness is key to suicide prevention. To date there is only limited evidence to support the efficacy of antidepressants in the prevention of suicide among depressed samples. Although the benefit of antidepressants in treating depression is well recognised, several studies have failed to support the efficacy of antidepressants in suicide prevention among depressed adults (Hirsch, 1982, Khan, 2003, Montgomery, 1983). Use of both antidepressants and psychosocial interventions may be a more promising means to prevent suicide. There is a need for greater coordination between general practitioners and allied health professionals in the treatment of high-risk individuals.

Depression's impact amongst older people is compounded by the fact that it sub-optimally diagnosed and treated (McCusker et al., 1998). There are several useful guidelines for the management of depression in older people (Curran et al., 2001, Baldwin et al., 2002a). Assessment tools are useful in screening (Watts et al., 2002), since they enable clinicians to systematically appraise the older person's status. A recent RCT found that screening for depression in long-term care residents increased the frequency of referral and treatment (Soon and Levine, 2002). There are a number of screening tools available (Pomeroy et al., 2001, Holtom and Barraclough, 2000, Lees and Lloyd-Williams, 1999). The Center for Epidemiological Studies Depression Scale (CES-D) and the Geriatric Depression Scale (GDS) (Radloff, 1977, Yesavage, 1983) are the two most widely used scales. The former has been used to identify depressive symptoms in epidemiological samples. The GDS is the commonest clinical screening tool, the 15 item version having the most psychometric testing. The GDS has good cross-cultural validity (Rait et al., 1999). There are a number of short screening tools that are useful in general practice, such as the two-item Patient Health Questionnaire (Li et al., 2007). Assessment tools, whilst valuable in detecting depressive symptoms, should be supported by efforts to obtain a greater understanding of the person's lived experience so as to be able to provide interventions that will best meet their individual needs.

A brief overview follows of the risk and protective factors associated with depression in older people. This knowledge can be used by older people and their formal and informal carers to aid the prevention of depression and assist in aspects of its management.

RISK AND PROTECTIVE FACTORS

Depressive symptoms are often key markers of broader aspects of emotional health and wellbeing. Working with an individual to address modifiable risk factors and to promote protective factors has the potential not only to improve depressive status, but also overall health and wellbeing.

Factors contributing to depressive symptomatology have been placed into three categories by Jorm and colleagues (Jorm, 2001):

1) Physical health
2) Stressful life events; and
3) Social health.

Compared to younger adults, the absolute risk of physical health problems and their associated effects upon independence via disability and handicap is significant amongst older individuals. Although older people have a propensity to develop resilience when faced with stressful life events, they are more likely to encounter key events such as the loss of a partner. These losses make them more vulnerable and can in turn influence their emotional health. Life changes are also pertinent to social health, the third category. A person's social connections are important to provide instrumental and emotional support and to maintain a sense of self-worth. An older person's social network may be diminished by bereavement, retirement and relocation.

RESIDENTS OF AGED CARE FACILITIES

Those living in institutionalised settings are at greater risk of depression. Depression is particularly prevalent amongst residents of aged care facilities, with rates of up to 50% reported (Baldwin et al., 2002a). In a study of depression incidence in those newly admitted to nursing homes in Australia, a quarter (24%) of the sample had major depression at one month post admission and a further 20% had a non-major depressive disorder (McSweeney and O'Connor, 2008). Rates were relatively stable at three and six-month follow-up. A small proportion (13%) showed symptom remission over the follow-up period. Crucially, major depression was only found in those with cognitive impairment (scores of 23 or less on the MMSE). The study is limited by its non-random sampling and 61% response rate, but the findings confirm those elsewhere in the literature highlighting that depression is an issue in aged care facilities (Teresi, 2001).

Depression amongst residents of aged care facilities is likely to be associated with the reduction in autonomy, independence, function and social support commonly experienced by residents. Moving to supported accommodation is a stressful life event. It can alter the person's social networks and lead to a reduction in emotional health. One only needs to consider the reasons for people to be admitted to see that the residents enter the accommodation with greater propensity to either have, or develop depression. Indeed, people living in supported accommodation are at greater risk for depression. In the Amsterdam Groningen Elderly Depression (AGED) study, a range of biological and psychological risk factors for depressive symptomatology were identified (Jongenelis et al., 2004). Prevalence amongst those in residential aged care facilities (RACFs) was three to four times higher that found in community dwelling counterparts. A multivariate logistic regression analysis found pain, history of stroke and visual impairment to be the key risk factors for depression in the 333 residents they assessed. Loneliness was the chief psychological risk factor. Being less than 80 years was also a significant risk factor. Systematic, ongoing assessment and monitoring of residents are therefore crucial. Communication with residents and their families is important. Staff need to explain how any illness is progressing. Residents need to be able to express how they are feeling without fear of censure. For example, a recent study discovered that residents felt reluctant to disclose feelings, for fear of being labelled a bad or weak person (Lloyd-Williams, 2002). This makes it difficult for aged care staff to pick up on depressive symptoms. An open, supportive environment that promotes trust can help overcome this barrier and assist the older person in making life transitions.

Recognition of depression in residents of aged care facilities, particularly those with dementia needs to be improved. The recognition of depression in dementia is challenging given the considerable overlap between depressive symptoms and those of dementia, and the increasingly impaired capacity of the dementia sufferer to reliably report depressive symptoms of depression (Draper, 1999). Comprehensive education regarding depression in dementia and training in the administration of scales such as the Cornell Scale for Depression in Dementia (CSDD) (Alexopoulos, 1998) have the potential to increase recognition and treatment rates greatly within nursing homes.

The management of nursing home residents with co-morbid depression and dementia requires more research. The evidence base to date suggests that for some residents with dementia, antidepressant medications may not prove to be effective in alleviating depression

(McSweeney and O'Connor, 2008). An alternative approach may be the use of psychosocial interventions. A recent review of the psychosocial treatment of depression in dementia (Teri, 2005) indicated that such interventions have the potential to improve depression greatly, even in the moderately to severely cognitively impaired. The interventions studied were performed in both community and institutional settings. The program components that appeared most effective were the individualization of strategies, using multiple treatment components, enhancing the communication and problem solving capacities of carers, and increasing the exposure of the depressed person to pleasant social interaction. A more recent systematic review of psychosocial treatments for psychological symptoms, including depression, in dementia sufferers confirms the paucity of evidence for such treatments (O'Connor et al., 2009). Music therapy and recreation therapy produced moderate effect sizes, but the extent of the duration of impact was not measured. More research is needed to enable refinement of techniques and to determine the characteristics of patients most suited to such interventions.

Prevention

Many interventions focus on managing the condition, but a more comprehensive, and potentially more successful approach is to prevent depression from occurring. Interventions to prevent depression have been found to be successful in a variety of studies. Cole and Dendukuri (2004) conducted a systematic review of brief interventions to prevent late life depression. They found 10 suitable studies with long-term follow up periods. There was general support for the feasibility of a range of interventions, including education and bereavement counselling. The impacts on depression risk were modest.

Management

There are four modes of management of depression: medical, psychological, lifestyle and alternative therapies. Some therapies are specific to depression, whilst others have broader health benefits. It is beyond the scope of this Chapter to review all the therapeutic evidence: a recent systematic review outlines the level of evidence for different antidepressant therapies that can be used with older people (Frazer et al., 2005). Amongst the psychotherapies, cognitive behaviour therapy and reminiscence and life review have the best supporting evidence for older people (Frazer et al., 2005, Jorm, 2002). Few lifestyle change modalities have been sufficiently tested to recommend their use with older people. An exception is physical activity. The following sections will discuss the evidence for antidepressant medications and physical activity, highlighting their advantages and disadvantages for older people. Finally, the importance of complementing any therapy with a balance diet will be noted.

ANTIDEPRESSANTS

Modern antidepressants are more targeted and have fewer side effects than their predecessors. They are an important means of managing major depression. They can be used to temper symptoms from the outset, enabling other therapeutic measures to be more readily adopted by the person.

There is level 1 evidence for the effectiveness of antidepressants in older people (Wilson et al., 2001). These findings apply across tricyclics, selective serotonin reuptake inhibitors (SSRIs) and monoamine oxidase inhibitors (MAOIs) and amongst community dwelling, institutionalised and hospitalised older people. The SSRIs are preferred for older people as they have fewer side effects than other groups. The serotonin and noradrenaline reuptake inhibitors (SNRIs) are effective, but the side effect profile is greater amongst frail older people.

Antidepressants benefit from ease of use. Nevertheless, antidepressant trials have reported high rates of adverse events (around 60%) (Salzman, 1993) and attrition (around 25%) (Mittman et al., 1997). Although most adverse events are mild and transient, for older people with depression side effects such as increased risk of hip fracture (Fiatarone Singh, 2002) need to be borne in mind when deciding treatment options. In older people, where other health problems are more likely to co-exist, there is the also likelihood of the adverse effects of polypharmacy. Depression can be a side effect of certain medications, such as some of those used in the management of arthritis (Leon et al., 2003). Given the risks of antidepressants, it is worth considering that for some people, such as those without major depression, non-pharmacological treatment may suffice. For others, use of adjunct therapies may enable the antidepressant dosage to be minimised.

PHYSICAL ACTIVITY

The following section considers the relationship between physical activity and depression. It explores potential underlying mechanisms for their association and reviews the evidence for the use of physical activity as an adjunct therapy in the management of depression. Depression often coincides with other health conditions. Ill health can lead to depression and depression can exacerbate other health problems. The impact of depression on stroke survivors will be used to illustrate this relationship. Physical activity's role in promoting other aspects of older people's health also will be highlighted. The potential risks of physical activity will be noted.

How Physical Activity Works

Whilst it remains unclear how exercise influences depression, several psychological and physiological mechanisms have been proposed (Lawlor and Hopker, 2001, Craft and Landers, 1998, Mather et al., 2002). Physical activity may provide distraction from negative thoughts. Physical activity is recognised as healthy lifestyle behaviour, so participants may experience positive feedback from others, improving their self esteem and self worth. For older adults adopting an exercise regime, there can be benefits from the mastery of a new skill. From a physiological perspective, in both animal models and depressed people, increased levels of neurotrophic factors in the brain following both exercise and antidepressant medication usage has been reported (Thornen et al., 1990, Duman, 2005). Exercise may also improve depression via social interaction.

The association between physical activity and depression

Prospective studies demonstrate that people who exercise are less likely to be- or become- depressed (Brosse et al., 2002). Cross-sectional and prospective studies of healthy adult populations have shown an association between physical inactivity and depression (Kritz-Silverstein et al., 2001, Lampinen et al., 2000, Moore et al., 1999, Lindwall et al., 2006) and indicate that a low prevalence of depressive symptomatology is related to exercise behaviour (Baldwin et al., 2002a, Blumenthal, 1999a, Lawlor and Hopker, 2001). Table 1 includes examples of studies that have investigated the relationship between physical activity and depression in older cohorts. Overall, results indicate that exercisers are less likely to have depressive mood, but to date the evidence that exercise protects against future depressed mood am Data from the Australian Longitudinal Study on Women's Health found that depression scores decreased and mental health scores increased with increasing levels of previous, current and habitual activity (Brown et al., 2005). Women who were active (one hour or more of moderate intensity activity per week) at baseline were 30 to 40% less likely to have poor mental health and depression scores than those less active. Those in the lowest category at baseline who became more active were also at lower risk of poor mental health scores than those who remained inactive. This association was independent of pre-existing physical or psychological health status.

In the Melbourne Longitudinal Studies on Healthy Ageing (MELSHA), both cross sectional and longitudinal analyses of the relationship between physical activity and depression have been conducted (Kendig et al., 1996) . Physical activity was measured in terms of both frequency and duration. Both baseline measures of physical activity were significantly negatively correlated with depressive status, measured using the depression subscale of the Psychogeriatric Assessment Scales (PAS-D) (-0.13 and -0.14 respectively). In further analyses, a range of demographic, health and lifestyle factors measured at baseline were used to determine univariate risk ratios for depression incidence two years later (Atlantis, 2009). The analyses excluded those classified as depressed at baseline. Chi square tests showed no significant difference in baseline physical activity frequency in those with depression (symptomatic or antidepressant use) compared to those without. Significant predictors of depression incidence were arthritis and respiratory disease, with prevalent gastrointestinal disease and increasing frequencies of self-reported pain also showing some association, suggesting that chronic disease and poor functional health were predictors of depression incidence at 2-year follow-up. There are various reasons for these conflicting results. The simplest is that during the intervening years, new and chronic health problems have led to the development of depression. There are also methodological bias issues related to self-reported assessment of physical activity and depressive status.ongst the non-clinically depressed remains equivocal.

Table 1. The association of physical activity and depression in selected cross-sectional and longitudinal studies

Author	Country	Sample size	Criteria	Odds Ratio/Effect size
Moore et al. 1999	USA	146, 50 years + Major depressive disorder	Minnesota Leisure-Time Physical Activity Questionnaire BDI	OR -0.17 (p = .045)
Brown et al. 2005	Australia	9207 women 45-55 years	CESD-10 SF-36 Mental health subscale Time spent in vigorous, less vigorous exercise, converted to MET mins	For high levels of physical activity (≥ 1200 or > 300 minutes/week) OR 0.62 for CESD-1- score ≥ 10 OR 0.55 for MH score ≤ 52
Lampinen et al. 2000	Finland	663, 65 years + 8 year follow up Physical activity behaviour categorised into necessary chores group, regular walking group and strenuous exercise group and change over time assessed in terms of maintained (stable), increased or decreased level (intensity) of physical activity	BDI-13 (Finnish version) Physical activity intensity- necessary chores, regular walking (at least weekly), strenuous physical activity Assessed changes in stability and intensity of physical activity over time	Depressive symptoms at follow-up predicted by necessary chores group: stable intensity 0.96 (NS) regular walking group: reduced intensity 10.56 stable intensity 2.21 (NS) strenuous exercise group: reduced intensity 1.23 (NS)
Kritz-Silverstein et al. 2001	USA	2029, 50-89 years 944 at 8 year follow up	BDI Regular strenuous exercise (Y/N), Exercise or labor at least three times/week (Y/N)	Only F tests reported
Lindwall et al., 2006	Sweden	860, 60 years + (mean 75.3, SD 10)	Montgomery Asberg Depression Rating Scale Frequency of light and strenuous intensity activity, change in last 12 months	Light exercise Never vs. every day d = 0.3 Never vs. no change d = 0.3 Strenuous exercise Never vs. every day d = 0.3 Never vs. no change d = 0.2

BDI = Beck Depression Inventory.

Physical Activity in the Prevention and Management of Depression

There is limited trial evidence for physical activity in the primary prevention of mental health problems. A review of interventions to *prevent* depression in older people did not include any physical activity trials (Cole and Dendukuri, 2004). To date, habitual physical activity has not been unequivocally shown to *prevent* the onset of depression.

However, there is growing evidence for the use of physical activity in the *management* of depression. Aerobic and resistance training have both produced benefits (Blumenthal, 1999a, Babyak et al., 2000, Singh et al., 1997, Singh et al., 2001, Singh et al., 2005, Stathopoulou et al., 2006). Both moderate and vigorous levels of exercise shows efficacy in reducing depressive symptoms (Dunn et al., 2001). Secondary analyses in an osteoarthritis trial found improvements in depressive symptoms and disability at 18 months post aerobic, but not resistance, training (Penninx et al., 2002). Even less intensive activity such as walking has been found to be effective (McNeil et al., 1991). Recent meta-analytic and experimental studies show a significant antidepressant effect for physical activity in older adults with

Table 2. Physical activity in the management of depression in older people : randomised trials with nonactive control conditions

Author	Sample	Intervention	Depression measurement tool	Outcome/Effect size
McNeil et al. 1991	30, mean age 72.5 years	Walking vs. social contact, waitlist control 6 weeks, no follow-up Attrition 0%	BDI	g 1.02
Singh et al. 1997	32, 60-84 years	PRT vs. health education 20 week program, 21 month follow-up Attrition 0%	BDI	g 1.76
Singh et al. 2005	60, 60-85 years	High intensity PRT vs. low intensity PRT, usual care 8 weeks, no follow-up Attrition 1%	HRSD	g 1.0
Sims et al. 2006	32, ≥ 65 years, mean age 74.3 years	PRT vs. waitlist control 10 weeks, 6 month follow up Attrition 6%	GDS, CES-D, PGMS	d 0.05, 10 weeks d 0. 07, 6 months

BDI = Beck Depression Inventory; CES-D = Center for Epidemiological Studies Depression Scale; GDS= Geriatric Depression Scale; HRSD = Hamilton Rating Scale for Depression; PGMS = Philadelphia Geriatric Morale Scale; PRT = progressive resistance training

g = Hedges (bias corrected) effect size; d = Cohen's effect size clinical depression, supporting the use of physical activity in the management of depression in older people (Taylor et al., 2004, Frazer et al., 2005). The Level 1 evidence suggests that physical activity is preferable to no treatment or social contact alone and that it has a similar effect to standard antidepressant drug or psychological treatments for both adults (North et al., 1990, Craft and Landers, 1998, Lawlor and Hopker, 2001, Brosse et al., 2002) and older adults (Palmer, 2005, Frazer et al., 2005). Reviewers have been critical of the quality of earlier studies (Lawlor and Hopker, 2001). Common methodological weaknesses include a lack of a standard diagnostic process for identifying depression in participants and a short follow up period (Lawlor and Hopker, 2001, Dunn et al., 2001). Table 2 provides examples of studies that have evaluated physical activity in the management of depression in older people with depressive symptoms.

Progressive Resistance Training

The evidence is particularly promising for progressive resistance training (PRT) (Lawlor and Hopker, 2001, Sjosten and Kivela, 2006, Barbour and Blumenthal, 2005). PRT offers an alternative form of physical activity for older people to aerobic physical activity. It has been particularly successful in ameliorating muscle weakness in older people. A decrease in muscle mass and muscle strength is a function of the ageing process, but can be exacerbated by chronic health problems. The weakness contributes to falls and fracture risk and overall disability. There has been substantial research that indicates PRT can improve muscle strength and physiological function. High intensity PRT is a safe, effective means to enhance muscle strength (Seynnes et al., 2004), assisting independence via functional and mobility improvements. In addition, by having a positive effect on bone health, PRT may reduce the potential for falling and osteoporosis.

Use of PRT to promote mental health appears to require high intensity activity to be effective. Singh and colleagues have reported positive effects following PRT in older people with depression. In 32 older people with depression, PRT significantly reduced Beck Depression scores compared to a group receiving health education, demonstrating that physical activity's therapeutic benefit was explained by more than socialisation (Singh et al., 1997). The impact is lasting: Singh and colleagues reported improvements in over 65 year olds' depression scores at 20 weeks (73% no longer depressed following high intensity PRT in a specialist clinic vs. 36% of controls receiving health education classes) (Singh et al., 2001). More recent research highlights the importance of exercise intensity, with a 50% reduction in depressive symptoms in most (61%) of their high intensity group compared to 29% in the low intensity group and 21% in the usual care group (Singh et al., 2005). The reduction was associated with actual strength gain, suggestive of an underlying biological mechanism. There were indications that vitality and sleep quality were particularly improved in the high intensity PRT group. Although social contact in exercise programs for older people with depression may contribute to the outcome, in Singh and colleague's research, the socialization at the exercise program did not seem to explain the impact of PRT: only the high intensity group achieved clinically significant benefits (Singh et al., 2005). Interestingly, belief in the perceived gains from the program seemed to produce a placebo effect for the low intensity group, whereas efficacy belief did not predict outcome in the high intensity group.

In contrast, elsewhere both high intensity and variable intensity PRT were found to improve measures of mood amongst sedentary, healthy older people (McLafferty et al., 2004). There were also gains in strength and lean body mass. Whilst many PRT programs have included healthy older people, benefits have also been seen for those with chronic disease e.g. osteoarthritis and chronic heart failure - and disability (Latham et al., 2005).

Although these trials provide support for PRT's use with older depressed people, translation of such evidence into routine practice has been limited. Access to specialist clinics and laboratories is less feasible for older people with mobility problems, or those living in rural and remote areas. The UPLIFT pilot study assessed the feasibility of older depressed people attending a community-based progressive resistance training (PRT) program (Sims, 2006). The randomised controlled trial also aimed to determine whether PRT improved depressive status in older depressed patients. People aged ≥ 65 years with depressive symptoms were recruited via general practices and randomly allocated to attend a local PRT program three times per week for 10 weeks or a brief advice control group. Depressive status, physical and psychological health, functional and quality of life status were re-assessed post intervention and at six months follow-up. Three hundred and forty six people responded to the study invitation, of whom 22% had depressive symptoms (GDS-30 score ≥ 11). A sample size of 130 was needed to detect a clinically significant (30%) group difference in depression rates, but unfortunately only 32 people entered the trial, so it was underpowered. There were no significant group differences on the GDS at follow-up. At six months there was a trend for the PRT group to have lower GDS scores than the comparison group, but this finding did not reach significance. More of the PRT group (57%) had a reduction in depressive symptoms post program, compared to 44% of the control group. It was not possible to discern which specific components of the program influenced its impact, but in post hoc analyses, improvement in depressive status was significantly associated with the number of exercise sessions completed (r = -0.8). Fifty eight percent met the adherence criterion of 60% or more sessions completed. This compares favourably with effectiveness studies, where participants attend a program at no cost and often with transport provided. There is scope for such a program to be offered by existing community-based facilities who have suitably trained exercise facilitators. More extensive implementation research will be needed to fully examine the effectiveness of such interventions when delivered in the community setting.

Other Forms of Physical Activity

Dance and movement therapy has been suggested as a potential means to reduce depressive symptoms. A therapist facilitates people to express themselves in movement and this is proposed to elevate mood. There are also potential benefits from the associated social interaction and listening to music. To our knowledge this therapy has not been evaluated in older adults. One study found that mood improved on the days the therapy occurred compared to other days, but no long term impact was assessed (Stewart et al., 1994) . Further research is required to assess the benefits.

Yoga exercises are popular and thought to promote well being. They may assist with the symptoms of stress and anxiety. There is modest, but limited evidence for yogic breathing exercises in adults. One study showed breathing exercises to be as effective as ADM for people with major depression, but less effective than electroconvulsive therapy

(Janakiramaiah et al., 2000). However, the researchers did not compare the intervention with placebo treatment.

The evidence arising from physical activity intervention trials needs to be interpreted with caution. Very few studies have ascertained clinical depression using DSM-IV criteria: they tend to focus on symptomatology, generally as measured using an assessment tool such as the GDS. Nevertheless, an improvement in symptomatology is valuable in its own right in promoting mental health and quality of life.

Physical Activity for Comorbid Conditions

Over half of older Australians are sedentary (Bauman, 2004). Given their absolute morbidity risk, sedentary older people have the potential to benefit from physical activity more than any other population sub-group. For older people with depression, physical activity may not only assist depression management: it can assist in the prevention and management of other health conditions.

There are many trials where people with a variety of conditions (e.g. coronary heart disease, chronic obstructive pulmonary disease, cancer, arthritis, multiple sclerosis, chronic fatigue syndrome), have demonstrated reduced levels of depressive symptoms following a physical activity program. Interpretation of these findings has to be sensitive not only to methodological constraints, but also to the fact that not all participants were clinically depressed at the time of the physical activity intervention (Paluska and Schwenk, 2000). To posit a clearer association, more studies using clinically depressed people are required.

Physical Activity for Co-Morbid Stroke

Impaired physical fitness can exacerbate disability in people with stroke. The use of physical activity with stroke patients has the potential to improve physical fitness and reduce disability. Coping with the functional impairments of a stroke may influence the onset of depression (Johnson, 1991). Depression is strongly linked with stroke, with comorbidity occurring in around 30% of people with stroke, adding to their disability (Burvill et al., 1995). Depression can therefore have a negative effect on rehabilitation and prognosis.

There is also evidence quality of life (QOL) is affected by stroke (Sturm and Donnan, 2004). People with depression after stroke display poorer social functioning (Clark and Smith, 1998) and poorer functional outcomes than non-depressed patients with stroke (Van de Weg et al., 1999). There has been little exploration of factors that potentially mediate these differences in recovery outcome. Whilst mobility benefits associated with exercise training have been documented (Saunders et al., 2004), there is a paucity of evidence supporting the influence of exercise therapy on post stroke depression or mental health (Morris et al., 2004), Two reviews of post stroke depression treatments failed to examine the use of physical activity (Kneebone and Dunmore, 2000, Whyte and Mulsant, 2002).

A Cochrane review of depression management in stroke patients found no evidence to support routine use of drugs or psychological therapies in this group (Hackett and Anderson, 2004). Whilst it is acknowledged that both therapies are helpful for adult depression, more information is needed on their use in people who have depression after stroke. This is particularly the case for antidepressant use, where there may be the risk of falls and a slight risk of seizures or delirium. As a non-drug treatment, exercise may be useful for stroke patients. Unlike psychotherapy it can impact directly on both mental and physical health. It may also reduce social isolation, a key risk factor for the development of depression after stroke (Ouimet et al., 2001).

The Regenerate study tested the feasibility of implementing a 10-week exercise intervention program for people experiencing clinically significant depressive symptoms post stroke (Sims et al., 2009). The aim of this randomised controlled trial was to examine whether PRT could reduce depressive symptoms and improve mental health, physical and social function, and quality of life amongst chronic stroke survivors. The PRT participants displayed significant improvements in upper and lower body muscle strength over the course of the exercise program, and several chose to continue with the program. However, the exercise group had lower depression scores than the controls at all time points, making an intervention effect difficult to discern. At 10-weeks follow-up, about half of both the exercise group and the control group demonstrated a reduction in their reported symptoms of depression. Twice as many of the exercise group had maintained these reductions at 6-months follow up, but this difference was no longer significant once baseline values were accounted for.

The second aspect of the Regenerate study aimed to examine factors that are associated with better quality of life in chronic stroke survivors 6 to 24 months post stroke (Teoh et al., 2009). Participants completed the study survey forms on three occasions over a six month period. The strongest predictors of post stroke quality of life were stroke severity and depressive status. People with less stroke severity and fewer depressive symptoms were more likely to experience good quality of life. The findings also suggested that being more optimistic, perceiving greater control over one's recovery and exercising regularly are also associated with better quality of life. It was clear that participants with few depressive symptoms following their stroke scored better on all quality of life, mental and physical health aspects of the surveys. Overall, there were significant improvements in participants' depressive status, physical health, emotional health, involvement in social activities and feelings of optimism over the 6-month course of the study. The findings highlight the important role that psychosocial factors play in chronic stroke survivors' quality of life. Targeting post-stroke depression and psychosocial adjustment to stroke within stroke rehabilitation programs has the potential to improve quality of life for chronic stroke survivors, independent of functional impairment. A range of health professionals, including psychiatrists, health psychologists, neurologists and geriatricians have an important role to play in managing the mental health and wellbeing of stroke survivors.

Physical Activity for Co-Morbid Dementia

This chapter has highlighted the greater rates of depressive symptomatology amongst those with dementia. There has been limited investigation of the use of physical activity to improve affect in this group. A recent randomised controlled trial compared a program of strength, balance and flexibility exercises with a supervised walking group and a social conversation control group (Williams, 2007). Ninety nursing home residents with Alzheimer's disease were randomly allocated to one of three groups that met for 15 minutes a day initially, increasing to 30 minutes later. Exercises included knee bends, toe rises and sidestepping plus walking. Walking group participants walked at their usual speed with support and rests as required. Conversation group members engaged in casual discussion of topics of mutual interest. Positive and negative affects were rated by blinded observers using the Alzheimer's Mood Scale (AMS) and the Observed Affect Scale (OAS) before and after the program. Ten weeks later, positive affect as measured by the OAS was significantly higher in the exercise group (15%) than the walking group and than the conversation group (9%). Negative affect scores on the AMS were significantly lower in the exercise group (12%) than the walking group and 21% lower than the conversation group. There were no significant differences for OAS negative affects or AMS positive affects.

SUMMARY

We know that anti-depressants and psychotherapies can assist in the management of depression. There is now growing evidence that physical activity can alleviate depression. In particular, progressive resistance training has been shown to be effective in managing major depression. In summary, many health benefits are associated with increased levels of physical activity in older people: lower rates of hypertension, heart disease, osteoporosis, degenerative arthritis, colonic cancer and diabetes mellitus, improved mood and memory function, and a better and maintained social network (Mazzeo and Tanaka, 2001).

Adherence to Treatment

No intervention is universally effective in the management of depression. Most therapies require to be used for some time before improvement is noted. Adherence is particularly important in the treatment of depression.

Current management of depression commonly involves drugs and psychotherapies, which whilst effective, have variable adherance rates. For some people adherence to physical activity may be easier than adherence to drug treatment. For others, adhering to physical activity regimes will also be challenging. The literature offers promising evidence of adherence amongst people with depression. For example, one study involving people who had not responded to antidepressant treatment (Mather et al., 2002) found that aerobic exercise was of short-term benefit as an adjunct treatment.

Depression has been associated with poor participation in physical activity and health promotion programs (McAuley et al., 1994), making it particularly critical to fully engage participants with depression in enjoyable activity to enable sustained benefits. In the Regenerate study, program adherence amongst stroke survivors with depression was good: on average 75% of the 10 week program was completed (Sims et al., 2009). Attrition was due to circumstances other than lack of motivation to attend. Long term adherence can be improved when the person makes physical activity part of their lifestyle (King, 1991). Some older people may prefer to exercise at home or on their own, for others joining a group based program can assist adherance via social interaction and the mutual commitment amongst participants (King et al., 1998).

Regular physical activity may also reduce the risk of depression relapse, although the evidence is scarce (Babyak et al., 2000). In a trial of older people with major depression, aerobic exercise was found to be of similar benefit to the antidepressant sertraline (Blumenthal, 1999b). At six months follow-up, relapse rates were lower in the exercise group (Babyak et al., 2000).

Risks of Physical Activity Participation for Older People

The risks associated with physical activity in older people are not too dissimilar from those for other adults. There are contraindications to physical activity, such as uncontrolled angina or blood pressure. Clinically these need to be addressed whether or not a person intends to be physical active and should only be temporary. The American College of Sports Medicine's 1998 Position Statement on Physical Activity in Older People (Mazzeo et al., 1998) reviewed the evidence for injury in trials and noted that no serious injury nor cardiovascular event has been reported. There have been isolated reports of minor injury e.g. tripping or sprains, but across the wealth of trials, reporting of adverse events has been rare; whilst this may be partly explained by publication bias, it is likely to reflect reality. For example, in an editorial, McMurdo refers to the exercise program run through the University of Dundee, Scotland. This program sees 1000 older participants per week on a self-referral, no screening, no disclaimer basis. Injuries are scarce. Commonly, modifications have been made to programs to ensure their suitability for people with pre-existing health problems, such as osteoarthritis. Overall, the risks of sedentary behaviour appear to outweigh those associated with physical activity.

Given this evidence, there has perhaps been undue cautiousness surrounding encouraging older people to be physically active. The fears possibly stemmed from the reports of adverse events associated with vigorous activity (as encouraged by previous guidelines). There is evidence from the Framingham Study that strenuous activity may be detrimental to older women's mortality rates (Sherman et al., 1994). Vigorous physical activity can increase the risk of sudden death, but the individual level risk is outweighed by the benefits (Bauman et al., 2002). The current Australian recommendations for older people advise beginning exercising gradually and with moderate intensity to promote safe physical activity (Sims et al., 2006).

Progression in physical activity intensity is vital. For older people starting or recommencing physical activity, beginning at a low intensity and gradually increasing to a moderate intensity will manage risk. Moderate intensity physical activity has greater potential to produce health benefits. The Australian National Heart Foundation guidelines for physical activity discuss indications for specific sub-groups of those with cardiovascular disease requiring medical clearance before commencing physical activity (Briffa et al., 2006). It is encouraging to note that across published chronic heart failure (CHF) trials, very few adverse events have been reported, no deaths or cardiac arrest and minimal orthopaedic injuries or serious arrhythmic events during training itself and few deaths during the studies (Witham et al., 2003). In a systematic review (Smart and Marwick, 2004) of 81 studies, representing 2387 people and more than 60,000 person-hours of physical activity there was no significant difference in the likelihood of deaths or adverse events between exercisers and controls with CHF during the trial period and an odds ratio of 0.71 for deaths in exercisers, indicating improved survival. These findings are particularly encouraging since many schemes have been conducted in the home, without telemetric monitoring.

Frail Older People

Older people are not to be excluded from physical activity solely on the basis of frailty. The American College of Sports Medicine's 1998 Position Statement on Physical Activity in Older People (Mazzeo et al., 1998) provided an overview of the evidence for physical activity adoption amongst frail older people. A growing number of studies have focused upon physical activity for older people in residential aged care facilities. Several of these are critiqued in a recent update of the literature (Cyarto et al., 2004). Unfortunately, many of the studies have had small sample sizes. An exception is a trial that involved 468 people which compared different types of physical activity programs for nursing home residents (Morris et al., 1999). In this cluster randomised trial, one group received mobility and strengthening program, another functional rehabilitation provided by nursing staff and the third received usual care. At 10 months follow up, there was a significant reduction in functional decline in the two intervention groups compared to the usual care group. In particular, declines in locomotion ability were noted. The intervention groups had a slight decline in GDS depression scores, but the difference was not significant. Participants GDS scores were relatively low: they were not clinically depressed, so the impact on depression cannot be determined from this particular study.

Nutrition and Depression Management

Management of the person with depression needs to be holistic and encompass the promotion of a balanced diet. The guidance notes underpinning the current Australian physical activity recommendations emphasise that physical activity adoption should be accompanied by a healthy balanced diet (Sims et al., 2006). This may be particularly important for older people with depression as there are physiological and behavioural links between diet and depression. Two potential pathways will be highlighted here, those involving homocysteine and cortisol respectively. Deficiencies in certain nutrients have been linked to depression, notably B group vitamins and folates. These nutrients are involved in the metabolic pathways that use amino acids methionine and homocysteine. These in turn contribute to the production and activation of neurotransmitters such as serotonin and dopamine. High levels of homocysteine have been implicated in the aetiology of depression. To date, the evidence for dietary supplementation is equivocal. Recent trials using folate, vitamin B6 and B12 supplementation have not markedly reduced risk (Ford et al., 2008). Ford et al (2008) showed no advantage of B vitamin supplementation compared to placebo over two years in reducing depression severity or incidence or promoting remission. There may be some genetic predisposition for raised homocysteine levels: supplementation may prove more helpful in individuals at higher risk. A meta-analysis reported that older people with high homocysteine levels had an increased risk of depression and that those with the methyltetrahydrofolate reductase (MTHFR) C677T genotype (TT) were 22% more likely than

CC carriers to have a history of depression or current depression (OR 1.22 95% CI 1.01-1.47) (Almeida et al., 2008). Homocysteine is also implicated in vascular health: lowered levels could contribute to prevention of cardiovascular disease, diabetes and dementia. Whilst there is insufficient evidence for dietary supplementation, ensuring that the individual does not have folate deficiency can protect against a range of health problems.

There is also emerging evidence for an association between certain forms of obesity and depression. Depression can raise cortisol levels, thereby raising blood glucose levels and influencing energy metabolism pathways. Cortisol activates lipoprotein lipase and inhibits lipid mobilisation, leading to fat deposition in the viscera. Low levels of sex steroid hormones (oestrogen and testosterone), also reported in depressed people, inhibits lipid mobilisation. Depression can also lead to people eating more energy rich 'comfort' foods, creating a similar scenario. Certain antidepressants, notably tricyclics, can also raise blood glucose. Dutch researchers recently reported an association between abdominal, visceral fat and depression in a prospective study of women aged 70-79 years (Vogelzangs et al., 2008). There was no association between depression and overall obesity, indicating a specific pathway. The association was significant for those depressed at baseline and for those experiencing recurrent bouts of depression.

Concluding Comments

Depressive illness results in considerable functional disability and decreased quality of life, particularly for older people. A range of approaches has been shown to improve depressive symptomatology. There is strong evidence for the use of antidepressants in the treatment of major depressive disorders. Non-pharmacological therapies such as psychotherapies and physical activity offer alternative or adjunct management of depression in older people.

Physical activity may assist both in the prevention and management of depression in older people. As a health promotion intervention, it has the potential to reduce the risk of depression and to ameliorate co-morbid conditions. Using physical activity as an antidepressant can reduce the need for pharmacological intervention, minimizing iatrogenic and polypharmacy risk that is particularly prevalent for older people.

Older depressed people have much to gain from being physically active. Physical activity offers a therapy where the adverse events are minimal and benefits can accrue for both physical and mental health status. For older people with depression, physical activity accompanied by a balanced diet may not only reduce depressive symptoms, but also improve overall health.

References

ALEXOPOULOS, G. S., ABRAMS, R. C., YOUNG, R. C., SHAMOIAN, C. A. (1998) Cornell Scale for Depression in Dementia. *Biological Psychiatry,* 23, 271-284.

ATLANTIS, E., GRAYSON, D, BROWNING, C, SIMS, J, and KENDIG, H. (2009) Cardiovascular disease and death associated with depression and antidepressants in the

Melbourne Longitudinal Study on Healthy Ageing (MELSHA) *Psychological Medicine*, Submitted.

AUSTRALIAN INSTITUTE FOR SUICIDE RESEARCH AND PREVENTION (2003) International Suicide Rates - Recent Trends and Implications for Australia. Canberra, Australian Government Department of Health and Ageing.

BABYAK, M., BLUMENTHAL, J. A., HERMAN, S., KHATRI, P., DORAISWAMY, M., MOORE, K., CRAIGHEAD, W. E., BALDEWICZ, T. T. and KRISHNAN, K. R. (2000) Exercise treatment for major depression: maintenance of therapeutic benefit at 10 months. *Psychosomatic Medicine,* 62, 633-8.

BALDWIN, R., CHIU, E., KATONA, C. and GRAHAM, N. (2002a) *Guidelines on depression in older people,* London, Martin Dunitz Ltd.

BALDWIN, R., CHIU, E., KATONA, C. and GRAHAM, N. (2002b) *Guidelines on depression in older people: practising the evidence,* London, Martin Dunitz Ltd.

BARBOUR, K. and BLUMENTHAL, J. (2005) Exercise training and depression in older adults. *Neurobiology of aging,* 26S, S119-S123.

BARRACLOUGH, J. (1997) ABC of palliative care: depression, anxiety and confusion. *British Medical Journal,* 315, 1365-1368.

BAUMAN, A. (2004) Health benefits of physical activity for older adults- epidemiological approaches to the evidence. IN MORRIS, M. and SCHOO, A. (Eds.) *Optimizing exercise and physical activity in older people.* Edinburgh, Butterman Heinemann.

BAUMAN, A., BELLEW, B., VITA, P., BROWN, W. and OWEN, N. (2002) Getting Australia active: Towards better practice for the promotion of physical activity. Melbourne, Australia, National Public Health Partnership.

BEEKMAN, A., COPELAND, J. and PRINCE, M. (1999) Review of community prevalence of depression in later life. *British Journal of Psychiatry,* 174, 307-311.

BEEKMAN, A. F., GEERLINGS, S., DEEG, D. and AL., E. (2002) The natural history of late-life depression. *Arch Gen Psychiatr,* 59, 605-611.

BLUMENTHAL, J. (1999a) The association between physical activity and depression in older depressed adults. *Journal of Ageing and Physical Activity,* 7, 55-61.

BLUMENTHAL, J. (1999b) The association between physical activity and depression in older depressed adults. *Journal of Aging and Physical Activity,* 7, 55-61.

BRIFFA, T. G., MAIORANA, A., SHEERIN, N. J., STUBBS, A. G., OLDENBURG, B. F., SAMMEL, N. L. and ALLAN, R. M. (2006) Physical activity for people with cardiovascular disease: recommendations of the National Heart Foundation of Australia. *Medical Journal of Australia,* 184, 71-75.

BROSSE, A. L., SHEETS, E. S., LETT, H. S. and BLUMENTHAL, J. A. (2002) Exercise and the treatment of clinical depression in adults: recent findings and future directions. *Sports Medicine,* 32, 741-60.

BROWN, W., FORD, J., BURTON, N., MARSHALL, A. and DOBSON, A. (2005) Prospective study of physical activity and depression in middle aged women. *American Journal of Preventive Medicine,* 29, 265-272.

BURVILL, P., JOHNSON, G., JAMROZIK, F., ANDERSON, C., STEWART-WYNNE, E. and CHAKERA, T. (1995) The prevalence of depression following stroke : the Perth Community Stroke Study. *Br J Psychiatry,* 166, 320-327.

CLARK, M. S. and SMITH, D. S. (1998) The effects of depression and abnormal illness behaviour on outcome following rehabilitation from stroke. *Clinical Rehabilitation,* 12, 73-80.

COLE, M. G. and DENDUKURI, N. (2004) The feasibility and effectiveness of brief interventions to prevent depression in older subjects: a systematic review. *International Journal of Geriatric Psychiatry,* 19, 1019-25.

CRAFT, L. and LANDERS, D. (1998) The effects of exercise on clinical depression and depression resulting from mental illness: A meta-regression analysis. *Journal of Sports and Exercise Psychology,* 20, 339-357.

CURRAN, J., WATTS, J. P. and LYNCH, S. (2001) Practical Management of Depression in Older People. London, Arnold.

CYARTO, E. V., MOORHEAD, G. E. and BROWN, W. J. (2004) Updating the evidence relating to physical activity intervention studies in older people. *Journal of Science and Medicine in Sport,* 7, 30-8.

DRAPER, B. M. (1999) The diagnosis and treatment of depression in dementia. *Psychiatric Services,* 50, 1151-1153.

DUMAN, R. (2005) Neurotrophic factors and regulation of mood: role of exercise, diet and metabolism. *Neurobiology of Ageing,* 26S, S88-S93.

DUNN, A., TRIVEDI, M. and AL., E. (2001) Physical activity dose-response effects on outcomes of depression and anxiety. *Medicine and Science in Sports and Exercise,* 33, S587-S597.

FIATARONE SINGH, M. A. (2002) Exercise in the oldest old: Some new insights and unanswered questions. *Journal of the American Geriatrics Society,* 50, 2089.

FRAZER, C. J., CHRISTENSEN, H. and GRIFFITHS, K. M. (2005) Effectiveness of treatments for depression in older people. *Medical Journal of Australia.,* 182, 637-32.

HACKETT, M. and ANDERSON, C., ET AL. (2004) Interventions for treating depression after stroke. *Cochrane Database of Systematic Reviews.* Chichester, UK., John Wiley and Sons Ltd.

HASIN, D., LINK, B. (1988) Age and recognition of depression:implications for a cohort effect in major depression. *Psychological Medicine,* 18, 683-688.

HENDERSON, A. S. (1994) Does ageing protect against depression? *Social Psychiatry and Psychiatric Epidemiology,* 29, 107-109.

HIRSCH, S. R., WALSH, C., DRAPER, R. (1982) Parasuicide. A review of treatment interventions. *Journal of Affective Disorders,* 4, 299-311.

HOLTOM, N. and BARRACLOUGH, J. (2000) Is the Hospital Anxiety and Depression Scale (HADS) useful in assessing depression in palliative care? *Palliative Medicine.,* 14, 219-20.

JANAKIRAMAIAH, N., GANGADHAR, B., NAGA, V., MURTHY, P., HARISH, M., SUBBAKRISHNA, D. and AL., E. (2000) Antidepressant efficacy of Sudarshan Kriya Yoga (SKY) in melancholia : a randomised comparison with electroconvulsive therapy (ECT) and imipramine. *J Affective Disorders,* 57, 255-259.

JOHNSON, G. A. (1991) Research into psychiatric disorder after stroke: the need for further studies. *Australian and New Zealand Journal of Psychiatry,* 25, 358-370.

JONGENELIS, K., POT, A., EISSES, A., BEEKMAN, A., KLUITER, H. and RIBBE, M. (2004) Prevalence and risk indicators of depression in elderly nursing home patients: the AGED study. *Journal of Affective Disorders.,* 83, 135-42.

JORM, A., CHRISTENSEN, H, GRIFFITHS, KM, ET AL. (2001) Help for depression: what works (and what doesn't). . Canberra, Centre for Mental Health Research.

JORM, A., CHRISTENSEN, H, GRIFFITHS, KM, RODGERS, B. (2002) Effectiveness of complementary and self-help treatments for depression. *Medical Journal of Australia.,* 176, S84-S96.

KENDIG, H., HELME, R., TESHUVA, K., OSBORNE, D., FLICKER, L. and BROWNING, C. (1996) *Health status of older people project: data report,* Melbourne, Victorian Health Promotion Foundation.

KHAN, A., KHAN, S.R., WALENS, G., KOLTS, R., GILLER, E.L. (2003) Frequency of positive studies among fixed and flexible dose antidepressant clinical trials: an analysis of the food and drug administration summary basis of approval reports. *Neuropsychopharmacology* 28, 552-557.

KING, A. (1991) Community intervention for promotion of physical activity and fitness. *Exercise and Sports Science Review,* 19, 211-260.

KING, A., RIJESKI, W. and BUCHNER, D. (1998) Physical activity interventions targeting older adults: a critical review and recommendations. *American Journal of Preventive Medicine,* 15, 316-333.

KNEEBONE, I. and DUNMORE, E. (2000) Psychological management of post-stroke depression. *British Journal of Clinical Psychology,* 39, 53-65.

KRITZ-SILVERSTEIN, D., BARRETT-CONNOR, E. and CORBEAU, C. (2001) Cross-sectional and prospective study of exercise and depressed mood in the elderly- the Rancho Bernardo Study. *American Journal of Epidemiology,* 153, 596-603.

LAMPINEN, P., HEIKKINEN, R. and RUOPPILA, I. (2000) Changes in Intensity of Physical Exercise as Predictors of Depressive Symptoms among Older Adults: An Eight-Year Follow-Up. *Preventive Medicine,* 30, 371-380.

LATHAM, N., ANDERSON, C., BENNETT, D. and STRETTON, C. (2005) Progressive resistance strength training for physical disability in older people. *Cochrane Database of Systematic Reviews.*

LAWLOR, D. and HOPKER, S. (2001) The effectiveness of exercise as an intervention in the management of depression: systematic review and meta-regression analysis of randomised controlled trials. *British Medical Journal,* 322, 763-767.

LEES, N. and LLOYD-WILLIAMS, M. (1999) Assessing depression in palliative care patients using the visual analogue scale: a pilot study. *European Journal of Cancer Care (Engl).* 8, 220-3.

LEON, F., ASHTON, A., D'MELLO, D., DANTZ, B., JEFFNER, J., MATSON, G. and AL., E. (2003) Depression and comorbid mental illness; therapeutic and diagnostic challenges. *Journal of Family Practice*, S19-S27.

LI, C., FRIEDMAN, B., CONWELL, Y. and FISCELLA, K. (2007) Validity of the Patient Health Questionnaire 2 (PHQ-2) in identifying major depression in older people. *Journal of the American Geriatric Society,* 55, 596-602.

LINDWALL, M., RENNEMARK, M., HALLING, A., BERGLUND, J. and HASSMEN, P. (2006) Depression and exercise in elderly men and women: findings from the Swedish National Study on Aging and Care. *Journal of Ageing and Physical Activity,* 15, 41-55.

LLOYD-WILLIAMS, M. (2002) Is it appropriate to screen palliative care patients for depression? *American Journal of Hospice Palliative Care.,* 19, 112-4.

MATHER, A., RODRIGUEZ, C., GUTHRIE, M., MCHARG, A., REID IC and MCMURDO, M. (2002) Effects of exercise on depressive symptoms in older adults with poorly responsive depressive disorder: Randomised controlled trial. *British Journal of Psychiatry,* 180, 411-415.

MAZZEO, R. S., CAVANAGH, P., EVANS, W. J., FIATARONE, M., HAGBERG, J., MCAULEY, E. and STARTZELL, J. (1998) Exercise and physical activity for older adults. *Medicine and Science in Sports and Exercise,* 30, 992-1008.

MAZZEO, R. S. and TANAKA, H. (2001) Exercise prescription for the elderly. *Sports Medicine,* 31, 809-818.

MCAULEY, E., COURNEYA, K., RUDOLPH, D. and LOX, C. (1994) Enhancing exercise adherence in middle-aged males and females. *Preventive Medicine,* 23, 498-506.

MCCUSKER, J., COLE, M. and KELLER, E. (1998) Effectiveness of Treatments of Depression in Older Ambulatory Patients. *Archives of Internal Medicine,* 158, 705-712.

MCLAFFERTY, C., WETZSTEIN, C. and HUNTER, G. (2004) Resistance training is associated with improved mood in healthy older adults. *Perceptual and Motor Skills,* 98, 947-957.

MCNEIL, J., LEBLANC, E. and AL., E. (1991) The effect of exercise on depressive symptoms in the moderately depressed elderly. *Psychology and Aging,* 6, 487-488.

MCSWEENEY, K. and O'CONNOR, D. (2008) Depression among newly admitted Australian nursing home residents. *International Psychogeraitrics,* 20, 724-737.

MITTMAN, N., HERRNANN, N., EINARSON, T., BUSTO, U., LANCTOT, K., LIU, B., SHULMAN, K., SILVER, I., NARANJO, C. and SHEAR, N. (1997) The efficacy, safety and tolerability of antidepressants in late life depression: a meta-analysis. *Journal of Affective Disorders,* 46, 191-217.

MONTGOMERY, S. A., ROY, D., MONTGOMERY, D.B. (1983) The prevention of recurrent suicidal acts. *British Journal of Clinical Pharmacology,* 15, 183s-188s.

MOORE, K. A., BABYAK, M. A., WOOD, C. E., NAPOLITANO, M. A., KHATRI, P., CRAIGHEAD, W. E., HERMAN, S., KRISHNAN, R. and BLUMENTHAL, J. A. (1999) The association between physical activity and depression in older depressed adults. *Journal of Ageing and Physical Activity,* 7, 55-61.

MORRIS, J., FIATARONE, M., KIELY, D., BELLEVILLE-TAYLOR, P., MURPHY, K., LITTLEHALE, S., OOI, W., O'NEILL, E. and DOYLE, N. (1999) Nursing rehabilitation and exercise strategies in the nursing home. *Journals of Gerontology. Series B, Psychological Sciences and Social Sciences* 54, M494.

MORRIS, S., DODD, K. and MORRIS, M. (2004) Outcomes of progressive resistance strength training following stroke: a systematic review. *Clinical Rehabilitation,* 18, 27-39.

NORTH, T. C., MCCULLAGH, P. and TRAN, Z. V. (1990) The effect of exercise on depression. *Exercise and Sports Science Review,* 18, 379-415.

O'CONNOR, D. (2006) Do older Australians truly have low rates of anxiety and depression? A critique of the 1997 National Survey of Mental Health and Wellbeing. *Australian and New Zealand Journal of Psychiatry,* 40, 623-631.

O'CONNOR, D., AMES, D., GARDNER, B. and KING, M. (2009) Psychosocial treatments of psychological symptoms in dementia: a systematic review of reports meeting quality standards. *International Psychogeraitrics*, 1-11.

OUIMET, M. A., PRIMEAU, F. and COLE, M. G. (2001) Psychosocial risk factors in poststroke depression: A systematic review *Canadian Journal of Psychiatry,* 46, 819-828.

PALMER, C. (2005) Exercise as a treatment for depression in elders. *Journal of the American Academy of Nurse Practitioners,* 17, 60-6.

PALUSKA , S. and SCHWENK, T. (2000) Physical activity and mental health: current concepts. *Sports Medicine,* 29, 167-180.

PEARSON, J. and BROWN, G. (2000) Suicide prevention in later life: directions for science and practice. *Clinical Psychology Reviews,* 20, 685-705.

PENNINX, B., REJESKI, W., PANDYA, J., MILLER, M. and AL., E. (2002) Exercise and depressive symptoms: A comparison of aerobic and resistance exercise effects on emotional and physical function in older persons with high and low depressive symptomatology. *Journals of Gerontology (B),* 57B, 24-132.

POMEROY, I. M., CLARK, C. R. and PHILLIP, I. (2001) The effectiveness of very short scales for depression screening in elderly medical patients. *International Journal of Geriatric Psychiatry,* 16.

RADLOFF, L. S. (1977) The CES-D scale: A self-report depression scale for research in the general population. *Applied Psychophysiological Measurement,* 1, 385-401.

RAIT, G., BURNS, A., BALDWIN, R. and AL., E. (1999) Screening for depression in African-Caribbean elders. *Family Practice,* 16, 591-595.

REGIER, D., BOYD, J., BURKE J and AL., E. (1988) One month prevalence of mental disorders in the United States. *Arch Gen Psychiatr,* 45, 977-986.

SABLE, J., DUNN, L. and ZISOOK, S. (2002) Late-life depression: how to identify its symptoms and provide effective treatment. *Geriatrics,* 57, 18-32.

SALZMAN, C., SCHNEIDER, L, LEBOWITZ, B. (1993) Antidepressant treatment of very old patients. *Am J Geriatr Psychiatry,* 1, 21-29.

SAUNDERS, D., GRIEG, C., YOUNG, A. and MEAD, G. (2004) Physical fitness training for stroke patients. (Cochrane Review). *The Cochrane Library.* Chichester, UK, John Wiley and Sons Ltd.

SAYER, G. P., BRITT, H., HORN, F., BHASALE, A., MCGEECHAN, K., CHARLES, J., MILLER, G. C., HULL, B. and SCAHILL, S. (2000) Measures of health and health care delivery in general practice in Australia. Canberra, Australian Institute of Health and Welfare and the University of Sydney.

SEYNNES, O., FIATRONE SINGH, M., HUE, O., PRAS, P., LEGROS, P. and BERNARD, P. (2004) Physiological and functional responses to low-moderate versus high-intensity progressive resistance training in frail elders. *Journal of Gerontology. Series A, Biological Sciences and Medical Sciences,* 59A, 503-509.

SHERMAN, S., D'AGOSTINO, R., COBB, J. and KANNELL, W. (1994) Does exercise reduce mortality rates in the elderly? Experience from the Framingham Heart Study. *American Heart Journal,* 128, 965-972.

SIMS, J., GALEA, M., TAYLOR, N., DODD, K., JESPERSEN, S., JOUBERT, J. and JOUBERT, L. (2009) Regenerate: assessing the feasibility of using a strength training program to enhance the physical and mental health of chronic post-stroke patients. *Int J. Geriatric Psychiatry,* 24, 76-83.

SIMS, J., HILL K, HUNT S, HARALAMBOUS, B., BROWN A, ENGEL L, HUANG N, KERSE N and M., O. (2006) National physical activity recommendations for older

Australians: Discussion document. A Report to the Department of Health and Ageing. April 2006. Melbourne, National Ageing Research Institute.

SIMS, J., HILL, K, DAVIDSON, S, GUNN, J, HUANG, N. (2006) Exploring the feasibility of a community-based strength training program for older people with depressive symptoms and its impact on depressive symptoms. *BMC Geriatrics.*

SINGH, N., CLEMENTS, K. and FIATRONE, M. (1997) A randomized controlled trial of progressive resistance training in depressed elders. *Journal of Gerontology,* 52A, M27-M35.

SINGH, N., CLEMENTS, K. and FIATRONE SINGH, M. (2001) The efficacy of exercise as a long-term antidepressant in elderly subjects: a randomised controlled trial. *Journal of Gerontology. Series A, Biological Sciences and Medical Sciences,* 50, M497-M504.

SINGH, N., STAVRINOS, T., SCARBEK, Y., GALAMBOS, G., LIBER C and FIATRONE SINGH, M. (2005) A randomized controlled trial of high versus low intensity weight training versus general practitioner care for clinical depression in older adults. *Journal of Gerontology. Series A, Biological Sciences and Medical Sciences,* 60A, 768-776.

SJOSTEN, N. and KIVELA, S.-L. (2006) The effects of physical exercise on depressive symptoms among the aged: a systematic review. *Int J Geriatric Psychiatry,* 21, 410-418.

SMART, N. and MARWICK, T. (2004) Exercise training for patients with heart failure: a systematic review of factors that improve mortality and morbidity. *American Journal of Medicine.,* 116, 693-706.

SNOW, V., LASCHER S and MOTTUR-PILSON, C. (2000) Pharmacological treatement of acute major depression and dysthymia. *Annals of Internal Medicine,* 132, 738-742.

SOON, J. and LEVINE, M. (2002) Screening for depression in patients in long-term care facilities: a randomized controlled trial of physician response. *Journal of the American Geriatric Society,* 50, 1092-9.

STATHOPOULOU, G., POWERS, M., BERRY, A., SMITS, J. and OTTO, M. (2006) Exercise interventions for mental health: a quantitative and qualitative review. *Clin Psychol Sci Pract,* 13, 179-193.

STEWART, N., MCMULLEN, L. and RUBIN, L. (1994) Movement therapy with depressed inpatients: a randomised multiple single case design. *Archives of Psychiatric Nursing,* 8, 22-29.

STURM, J. and DONNAN, G., ET AL (2004) Quality of life after stroke: The North East Melbourne Stroke Incidence study (NEMESIS). *Stroke,* 35, 2340-2347.

TAYLOR, A. H., CABLE, N. T., FAULKNER, G., HILLSDON, M., NARICI, M. and VAN DER BIJ, A. (2004) Physical activity and older adults: a review of health benefits and the effectiveness of interventions. *Journal of Sports Sciences,* 22, 703-725.

TEOH, V., SIMS, J. and MILGROM, J. (2009) Psychosocial predictors of quality of life following a stroke. *Topics in Stroke Rehabilitation*, in press.

TERESI, J., ABRAMS, R., HOLMES, D., RAMIREZ, M., EIMICKE, J. (2001) Prevalence of depression and depression recognition in nursing homes. *Social Psychiatry and Psychiatric Epidemiology,* 36, 613-620.

TERI, L., MCKENZIE, G., LAFAZIA, D. (2005) Psychosocial treatment of depression in older

adults with dementia. *Clinical Psychology: Science and Practice,* 12, 303-316.

THORNEN, P., FLORAS, J., HOFFMAN, P. and SEALS, D. (1990) Endorphins and exercise: physiological mechanisms and clinical implications. *Med Sci Sports Exerc,* 22, 417-428.

VAN DE WEG, F. B., KUIK, D. J. and LANKHORST, G. J. (1999) Post-stroke depression and functional outcome: a cohort study investigating the influence of depression on functional recovery from stroke. *Clinical Rehabilitation,* 13, 268-272.

VOGELZANGS, N., KRITCHEVSKY, S., BEEKMAN, A., NEWMAN, A., SATTERFIELD, S., SIMONSICK, E., YAFFE, K., HARRIS, T. and PENNINX, B. (2008) Depressive Symptoms and Change in Abdominal Obesity in Older Persons *Arch Gen Psychiatry,* 65, 1386-1393.

WATTS, S., BHUTANI, G., STOUT, I., DUCKER, G., CLEATOR, P., MCGARRY, J. and DAY, M. (2002) Mental health in older adult recipients of primary care services: is depression the key issue? Identification, treatment and the general practitioner. *International Journal of Geriatric Psychiatry.,* 17, 427-37.

WHYTE, E. and MULSANT, B. (2002) Post stroke depression: epidemiology, pathophysiology and biological treatment. *Biological Psychiatry,* 52, 253-264.

WILLIAMS, C. L., TAPPEN, R. M. (2007) Effect of exercise on mood in nursing home residents with Alzheimer's disease. *American Journal of Alzheimer's Disease and Other Dementias,* 22, 389-397.

WILSON, K., MOTTRAM, P., SIVANRANTHAN, A. and A., N. (2001) Antidepressants versus placebo for the depressed elderly. The Cochrane Database of Systematic Reviews.

WITHAM, M. D., STRUTHERS, A. D. and MCMURDO, M. E. (2003) Exercise training as a therapy for chronic heart failure: can older people benefit? *Journal of the American Geriatrics Society,* 51, 699-709.

YESAVAGE, J., ET AL. (1983) Development and validation of a geriatric depression screening scale: a preliminary report *Journal of Psychiatric Research,* 17, 37-49.

In: Psychiatric Research Trends: Dreams and Geriatric Psychiatry ISBN 978-1-60741-760-6
Editors: Daniella M. Montez, pp.27-45

Chapter 2

HOW TO SECURE THE FUTURE OF THE MENTAL HEALTH OF FAMILIES IN CHARGE OF THEIR ELDERS

Stephanie Carretero*[1]*, Jorge Garcés and Francisco Ródenas
Polibienestar Research Institute, University of Valencia, Spain

ABSTRACT

The burden or stress of the informal carer of dependent elderly people is nowadays one of the main mental health problems, mainly due to the increasing number of elderly people in need of care and help from others in the developed countries. The informal caregiver burden affects especially middle-aged women, who are the typical profile of the person in charge of old dependent adults. These women are affected mainly by depression, anxiety and high stress level and of course use a higher number of psychotropic medicines.

Negative impact on physical health also exists such as negative evaluations of their own health, psychosomatic and immunological disorders, cardiovascular problems, and dependency in order to perform the activities of daily life. The caregiver burden, the emotional discomfort, and indicators of the poor state of health also appear as major predictors of the premature institutionalization and mistreatment of the care recipient.

The results of the research, guided in the majority of cases by the theoretical framework of Pearlin by means of his Stress Process Model (Pearlin et al., 1989, 1990; Pearlin, 1991) has determined the choice for the study of the determining variables of the informal caregiver burden. In this sense, scientific thought shows the existence of multiple variables associated with the caregiver burden, among which it is possible to highlight, in Pearlin's terms, that the variables of the care context as well as the primary stress factors comprise a primary generator core of the burden, whereas the secondary stress factors represent the proliferation of the emotional discomfort and burden in other areas of life.

Our research has indicated that the psycho-educational intervention programs framed within the respite services jointly with the knowledge of the determining variables of the burden can comprise the best optimal approach in order to effectively deal with the

---

[1] Corresponding Author. Dr Stephanie Carretero. Address: ERI Polibienestar, Universitat de València. Avda de los naranjos, s/n. 46022 Valencia (Spain). Tel: +34963828184, Fax: +34063828188. Email:stephanie. carretero@uv.es.

burden problem of the informal caregivers of dependent senior citizens. Regarding this, this chapter reviews the main theories and results of the existing research to date about the concept of the informal caregiver's burden. The explanation of the burden concept, the theoretical approaches which attempt to explain it, the variables which have emerged in the investigation, the predictors of its appearance, as well as the intervention programs developed to relieve the burden, in order to allow us to approach the appropriate solutions to deal with the current social and political reality of this problem.

1. Introduction

Europe and the U.S.A. are currently facing demographic aging with equivalently high rates of senior citizens (Vevren, 2006) and, consequently, an increase in their dependent population—where dependency is understood as the state in which a person requires the help of others in order to perform daily activities (Council of Europe, 1998). The informal care is the assistance provided by persons from the intimate environment of the dependent person (family, neighbors, and friends), who do not possess any training about care and who do not receive any economic retribution for this task. The in-home care provided by informal caregivers, especially by family members, is due to different reasons—the preference of the affected patients to remain in their residence, the high cost of formal resources, and the family-oriented character of Mediterranean society, being the most frequent. Consequently, the majority of the long-term care burden of dependent people falls upon the informal caregivers.

Thus, there are approximately 5% of European informal caregivers of dependent people which are dedicated to informal care (INE, 2004). The informal caregivers are usually family members, normally female—wife or daughter—between the ages of 45 and 65, without job employment or with part-time employment and a low educational and socio-economic level. Additionally, the care provision is usually characterized by being supplied in the residence of the dependent person—a house which is often shared—in a continual, intense, and daily way (which can represent over 40 hours a week), and includes diverse types of services which range from personal care and the performance of domestic tasks to emotional support. Generally, this assistance is assumed by a single caregiver; a responsibility which frequently lasts for years, where findings show a weighted average of approximately 5 years for dependent people in different environments (Family Caregiver Alliance, 2001; Carretero et al. 2007).

Having outlined this situation, it is not surprising from the Psychology perspective that there is a major concern regarding the impact of the care situation of a dependent person which can be generated on the informal caregiver. In this sense, informal care has been conceptualized as a vital stress factor event (Zarit, 2002), which jointly with its chronicity and the lack of foresight about the time of its finalization, have been associated with negative repercussions on the physical and psychological well-being of the informal caregiver. This situation has been generically denominated with the overall term of *caregiver burden.*

Moreover, the care burden is not only a social and health problem but also an economic and political one in the financial pressure it causes on the social protection systems. On the one hand, carers' own health problems resulting from the care burden may convert them too into consumers of the health system, thus adding to the pressure of the dependants' need for health care (Havens, 1999). On the other, when the informal sector becomes overburdened, the demand for long-term care moves to the public and private institutional sector. All of this creates a political, health, social and economic problem if we consider the current loss of sustainability of social protection systems (Garcés, Ródenas and Sanjosé, 2003).

As a result, we have performed the following theoretical and empirical revision of the burden concept and the intervention programs developed which will make it possible to inform and orient the Public Administrations and, in turn, it will serve as a guide for researchers and professionals involved in the responsibility to handle the problems linked to the burden of the informal caregivers of senior dependent people.

2. The Burden Concept: Theoretical Perspectives about Caregiver Stress

At the beginning of the 1960s, Grad and Sainsbury (1963) mentioned this concept for the first time in the scientific bibliography, when they described the burden perceived by family members when caring for their relatives, affected by some mental illness, in their residence. The definition which was given to the burden concept at that time, and which has been adopted by other authors in a more or less extensive way in the research about the negative repercussions of informal care, has been to assume it as an overall term in order to describe the physical, emotional, and economic consequence of providing care (Mockus Parks and Novielli, 2000; Gaugler et al., 2000).

In this sense, it is worth highlighting the contributions made by Zarit and collaborators who identified the burden generated by the provision of care as "a state resulting from the action of taking care of a dependent or elderly person, a state which threatens the physical and mental health of the caregiver" (Zarit et al., 1980), as well as by George and Gwyther who understood burden as "the persistent difficulty to provide care and the physical, psychological, and emotional problems which caregivers or family members can experience when caring for a relative with a disability or some type of deterioration" (George and Gwyther, 1986). Similarly, other authors have described burden as the impact that care has on mental health, physical health, other family relations, the job, and the financial problems of the caregiver (Pearlin et al., 1990; Gaugler et al., 2000).

In spite of the multiple investigations performed in the last three decades, above all in the field of family caregivers of ill patients affected by some dementia such as Alzheimer's disease, the caregiver's burden continues to be an ample term with many definitions; in this respect, there is still no homogeneity in relation to its meaning and use (Friss, 2002).

In an attempt to define the burden in a more specific and detailed way, a differentiation has been made between objective and subjective components, which has given rise to the concepts of subjective and objective burden (Montgomery et al., 1985). In fact, this distinction obeys the specific development of the burden concept and points to the multidimensionality of the impact of care (Montgomery and Borgatta, 1989). Thus, in the first moment, the burden term was elaborated as a subjective perception of the impact of care by the caregiver, where subjective burden refers to the attitudes and emotional reaction of the caregiver faced with the development of the care, such as for example, a low emotional mood, anxiety, or depression. Subsequently, the objective component of the burden was included, which related the objective burden with the dedication to the fulfillment of the caregiver role and involved the specific repercussions on the different areas of the caregiver's life—employment, social life, leisure, etc.—(Montgomery, 1989; International Psychogeriatric Association, 2002).

Nonetheless, research has demonstrated that the caregiver burden cannot be summarized in a unique concept, which encompasses multiple dimensions, subject to individual variability and whose process of adaptation fluctuates throughout the care period (Zarit, 2002). They comprise the main reasons why it has been defended that the caregiver burden must be framed within a multi-dimensional process, where different explanatory theoretical models have appeared from Psychology regarding the complexity of the caregiver burden.

Basically, from the theoretical viewpoint, the burden has been explained from the psychological perspectives of stress and coping (Gaugler, et al., 2000). Specifically, the majority of theoretical models which have been developed to explain the burden and the stress of the caregiver have been based on the Transactional Stress Theory by Lazarus and Folkman (1984). In this context, the model which has had the greatest influence in the theoretical understanding of the process of the caregiver burden has been the *Pearlin Stress Process Model* (Pearlin et al., 1989; Pearlin et al., 1990; Pearlin, 1991; Aneshensel et al., 1995; Pearlin and Skaff, 1995). The authors assume a multi-dimensional approach to describe how the care is converted into a burden for some individuals and can lead to physical and psychological reactions in the caregiver.

Specifically, Pearlin and his collaborators defend the influence of the *contextual characteristics* of the caregiver and the recipient of the care – for example, sociodemographic variables – in the caregiver's adaptation to the stress process of the care. Furthermore, they propose that there are various types of stress factors which determine the caregiver burden. In this sense, they affirm that the care demands (*objective primary stress factors*) have a repercussion on the caregivers provoking a series of negative emotional reactions (*the subjective primary stress factors*) in them.

The primary stress factors can in turn proliferate in other areas of the caregiver's life (*secondary stress factors*) and in an objective way, provoke negative repercussions on the free time, social relations, the economic and employment situation of the caregiver (role tensions) and the subjective assessment of these consequences can lead to diminished feelings of self-esteem, expertise, sense of self, or competency (intrapsychic tensions). The stress process can be mediated by variables that mitigate the negative impact of the care implications which *include strategies of coping and social support,* both formal and informal, which alleviate the stress and the negative mental health associated to the care task.

Zarit has expanded this model, including in a successive way, the secondary assessments – *Expanded Theoretical Model of Care* (Zarit, 1989, 1990) – and primary assessments – *Modified Stress Process Model of Lazarus and Pearlin* (Zarit, 2002) – from the theory of Lazarus and Folkman (1984) which, applied to the care context, imply in a respective way, that the caregiver makes a general assessment of his/her own resources in order to confront the threat of the stress factors of the care as well as a subjective evaluation of the objective primary stress factors in terms of threat or challenge.

These theoretical approaches have not ceased to confirm what we have already mentioned above: The multi-dimensionality of the process of the informal caregiver's burden. The revision of the research conducted in this respect equally denotes the multiple variables associated to the caregiver's burden, as well as the different repercussions on the physical and mental well-being of the care.

3. Empirical Results about Caregiver Stress

The studies have shown that the *existence of negative repercussions of the burden on the physical and mental health* of the informal caregivers of dependent people. On one hand, the effects of the caregiver burden on the *mental health* of the caregivers are essentially depression and anxiety as well as high stress levels; equally it finds that the probability of the development of these disorders is greater in women than in men, and this larger risk is also linked with a greater assumption of responsibility in the caregiver task , a greater number of hours providing the care, and a greater physical and cognitive deterioration of the care recipient (Yee and Schulz, 2000). Equally, it is worth noting that the greater incidence of mental health disorders is corroborated by the greater use of psychotropic medicine among the caregivers in comparison with the general population (Noonan and Tennstedt, 1997).

Among the effects on *the physical health*, although less frequent and intense than the aforementioned effects on the mental health, we find: negative evaluations of their own health, psychosomatic and immunological disorders, cardiovascular problems, and dependency in order to perform the activities of daily life. Equally, it has found that the caregivers neglect their own health needs, thus they have a lower probability to become involved in preventive health behaviors and to seek medical care These problems generate an increased risk of premature mortality in the caregivers (Lee et al., 2003; Grunfeld et al., 2004).

The caregiver's burden can also lead to major negative consequences for the dependent person, which include *premature institutionalization and mistreatment.* On the one hand, the caregiver burden, the emotional discomfort, and indicators of the poor state of health appear as major predictors of the abandonment of the care task and the consequent institutionalization of the dependent person as opposed to the variables of the dependent person- evolution of the disease, behavior problems, cognitive alterations, difficulties in the performance of the daily activities - (Logdon et al., 1999).

Nevertheless, according to the Pearlin Stress Process Model - in which the caregiver burden has been conceptualized as a process – the institutionalization does not represent a solution for the care burden: the entry of a dependent person in a center leads to the disappearance of specific stress factors associated with the in-home care period but the appearance of others linked to the institutional care. In addition, the stress developed in the in-home care phase continues to have an influence in the institutional care phase (Pearlin et al., 1990; Pearlin, 1990; Aneshensel et al., 1995; Pearlin and Skaff, 1995).

It has also indicated that the caregivers can be involved in aggressive or violent behaviors towards the caregiver as a consequence of the burden that he/she is experiencing, by means of mistreatment or abuses (Havens, 1999; Mockus Parks and Novielli, 2000).

Several authors have also appealed to the possibility of the existence of *positive repercussions of care* (Marks et al., 2002), where several investigations have indicated an increase of expertise and the feelings of satisfaction derived from caring for a dependent person as the two most relevant positive consequences.

On the other hand, from the empirical viewpoint, multiple investigations have been carried out to identify the variables associated with the caregiver burden, which highlight the following:

Among the *variables of the care context,* a series of sociodemographic characteristics of the caregiver and the caregiver – care recipient relation, are associated to the burden levels of the care provider.

Specifically, among the sociodemographic variables of the caregiver, a young age, being a female, a low income level of the caregiver and the fact that this person has a job have been associated with very high levels of burden (Navaies-Waliser et al., 2002).

Equally, with regards to the *relation between the caregiver and the care recipient,* variables appear which are more intensely related to the caregiver burden: the family relation and whether or not the day caregiver lives with the patient. Spouses experienced greater levels of excessive burden than the children of dependent people (International Psychogeriatric Association, 2002), essentially due to the greater physical and emotional closeness of the couples (Gaugler et al., 2000), although it is also necessary to consider in this case, the influence of the gender variable since the daughters and the wives experience similar levels of burden greater than those shown by the sons and the husbands who are caregivers (Hawranik and Strain, 2000). The fact that the caregiver lives with the dependent person is related to high levels of excessive burden, depression, social isolation, and poor state of health, primarily generated by the greater daily frequency of the care and the greater commitment to maintain the person in the residence (Brodaty and Hadzi-Pavlovic, 1990; International Psychogeriatric Association, 2002).

We also note that few studies have been carried out in relation to the *sociodemographic variables of the dependent person,* essentially given the fact that when it has been desired to analyze the influence of the characteristics of the care recipient on the caregiver burden, the majority of the research have preferred to focus on the factors associated to the dependence and the disease - which means, the objective primary stress factors –. Only a few researchers have indicated in a very general way that a young age and the male gender of the care recipient can be related to a greater caregiver burden (Gaugler et al., 2000).

With regard to the *primary stress factors*, the influence of behavioral problems generated by dementias or other mental disorders can appear in a severe way – as opposed to the cognitive deficiencies and dependence for the activities of daily life, as generators of excessive burden in the caregiver, emotional discomfort, exhaustion, and emotional mood disorders (Dunkin and Anderson-Haley, 1998; Hawranik and Strain, 2000).

In the case of the absence of any mental pathology, the dependency for the activities of daily life, the progressive physical deterioration, and the amount of activities for which the person is dependent, appear strongly related to the caregiver burden (Logsdon et al., 1998; Gaugler et al., 2000).

Both the behavioral and functional problems have been linked to the excessive burden of the role, although over time, the behavioral problems are the only ones that are associated with this subjective primary stress factor (Aneshensel et al., 1995; Gaugler et al., 2000). It has been indicated that perhaps the relevancy in the prediction of the caregiver burden is due to the unpredictability and irregularity of the demands. The behavioral problems are not foreseeable nor of regular appearance, as opposed to the characteristics of the disease and the dependency which appear in a more systematic way and are assumed in a more natural way in the caregiver role (Deimling and Bass, 1986; Gaugler et al., 2000).

In relation to the *secondary stress factors,* the impact of the care situation causes the multiplication or proliferation of emotional discomfort and an excessive burden on other areas of the caregiver's life. The repercussions are diverse and can become evident in the form of a reduction of free time, leisure activities, social relations, appearance of family and matrimonial conflicts (Semple, 1992; Aneshensel et al., 1995).

We also highlight the problems which appear in the employment environment such as: quitting the job, reduction or readjustment of the workday hours, impossibility to access the job market, increases in the workday hours to compensate the loss of income provoked by the care, loss of incomes and negative effects on promotion and job ascent (Havens, 1999; Jenson and Jacobzone, 2000). The possibility of the appearance of these effects increases with a longer period of care, with the greater seriousness of the illness, if the caregiver is a woman as well as an elderly age (Mears, 1998).

The care also has an economic repercussion on the caregiver. In particular, there is a tendency to lose acquisitive power caused by the reduction of the incomes derived from work, as well as those derived by the cost generated by the specific care requirements for the dependent person (Grunfeld et al., 2004).

On the other hand, the caregiver burden can be alleviated by means of two types of *mediators:* the strategies of coping and social support. It has been indicated that the strategies focused on the problem (such as problem solving or the redefinition of the care situation) are more effective to alleviate the effects of the caregiver burden and in the reduction of the psychological discomfort than those focused on emotion (Pearlin and Skaff, 1995; Mockus Parks, and Novielli, 2000). Nevertheless, it has been defended that this relation is complex and that the different strategies of confrontation have effects based on the phase of the care process in which the caregiver is found, on different emotions, and according to the primary stress factor involved. Specifically, the expertise will only be effective during the in-home care, not during the institutionalization phase, while the strategies of confrontation focused on the problem will be effective to increase the positive effect and those focused on emotion as reducers of the emotional discomfort - depression and anxiety - (Aneshensel et al., 1995).

Social support has appeared as another mediator variable of the stress process, either by means of the informal system or the formal resources. In this sense, the investigation results indicate that the assistance of an instrumental and/or emotional type supplied by family members and neighbors to the informal caregiver is efficient, respectively, to reduce the excessive burden and improve the well-being (Markus Parks and Novielli, 2000). Although, these positive effects on the caregiver burden can be eclipsed by the presence of family conflicts (Semple, 1992; MaloneBeach and Zarit, 1995).

Equally, the relief addressed to caregivers provided by the formal resources has been the object of research, especially the respite services and psychosocial intervention programs. The main advantages of these resources is their capacity to reduce the caregiver burden, the tension, and emotional discomfort as well as the negative consequences on the different areas of the caregiver's life, and on the other hand, they make it possible to fulfill the preferences of the dependent person to remain in his/her house and the community in order to receive long-term care, which in fact, is associated with a greater quality of life, well-being, and longevity (Havens, 1999).

4. Intervention Programs to Alleviate the Caregiver Burden: The Respite Services and Psychosocial Programs

4.1. Respite Services

The research on interventions to reduce the carer burden has focused above all on the programmes that use formal services to allow the dependent person to remain in the community, based on the available evidence that both the families and members of informal networks caring for dependent persons and the dependants themselves prefer to remain in their homes and in their community receiving long-term care (Havens, 1999) and that remaining at home has been linked to greater longevity and quality of life for the dependent person (Bowers, 1987). The formal support services to alleviate carer burden that have received most attention as specific intervention programmes are *respite services* (Zarit, Gaugler and Jarrot, 1999; International Psychogeriatric Association, 2002).

The purpose of formal respite programmes is to relieve carers periodically or temporarily from their responsibility and from the provision of care for their dependants. This rest allows the carer to spend some time alone and carry out other activities or deal with other obligations (Whittier, Coon and Aaker, 2002).

Studies have shown that intervention in the form of respite services affects the carer's wellbeing by alleviating or reducing the burden (Zarit, 1990b; Fernández-Ballesteros and Díez, 2001; Whittier, Coon and Aaker, 2002). They therefore help the informal carer to continue providing care in the home and avoid early institutionalisation of the dependant (International Psychogeriatric Association, 2002; Whittier, Coon and Aaker, 2002). Also, such services allow care recipients to improve their behavioural problems, health, state of mind, satisfaction with life and wellbeing (Zarit et al., 1999).

There are three types of respite service available to relieve carer stress: 1) home help; 2) day centre; and 3) residential or night-time respite.

In general, *home help* is when periodic assistance is received for caring for the dependant with a specific duration, allowing the main carer to leave the home or carry out other tasks (Havens, 1999; Whittier, Coon and Aaker, 2002). Examples of the type of care provided by the home help services are housework, physical care, supervision and accompanying the dependant, etc. (Zarit, Gaugler and Jarrot, 2000).

Day centres allow the dependent person to go during the day to a supervised, structured centre where social and health care can be provided, freeing the carer for other activities or rest (Zarit et al., 1999; Kropf, 2000; Zarit, 2002). This is a type of collective or group home help that facilitates social contact for the dependant person who is generally isolated from the community (Watanabe et al., 1994).

Residential or night-time respite care involves the admission of the dependent person in a residence, hospital or other type of institutional centre for long-term care for the full 24 hours over a period that may vary between one night to several weeks depending on the needs of the main carer (Havens, 1999; Whittier, Coon and Aaker, 2002).

The negative effects of respite services on care have been the subject of several research studies. Temporary institutionalisation is perhaps the resource that has been studied least and the way it ties in with the care burden is not altogether clear (Whittier, Coon and Aaker,

2002). The studies have shown that this type of respite service can reduce the carer's physical and mental burden, but only providing temporary relief (Zarit et al., 1999).

Home help and day centres, on the other hand, have appeared more frequently in the literature as being significantly associated with greater physical and psychological wellbeing for the carer. The research has shown that carers who use such respite services suffer lower levels of perceived stress, burden, anxiety and depression, fewer somatic illnesses, less anger and more positive feelings (Lyons and Zarit, 1999; Zarit et al., 1999; Hawranik and Strain, 2000; Zarit, 2002). This type of assistance has also been related with lower degrees of social and emotional isolation for the carer and higher levels of self-esteem, assertiveness, control over their own lives (Bourgeois, Schultz and Burgio, 1996) and general satisfaction (Lawton, Brody and Saperstein, 1989). It has been found that this greater wellbeing for carers is due to the fact that both these resources, especially day centres, allow them to organise the caring time and reduce the time that the care recipient is alone, both substituting and complementing the informal care. Carers with a job are able to pass over care to a formal resource for a longer number of hours and days (Jarrot and Zarit, 1995).

In spite of the above, the link between the use of formal social resources and the decreasing carer burden is still complex, especially because: a) the use of formal respite services has also been linked to greater tension and depression for the carer (Morris, Morris and Britton, 1989), persistence of depression symptoms (Lyons and Zarit, 1999; Zarit et al., 1999; Hawranik and Strain, 2000), greater family conflict as a result of disagreements about the services to be received and/or the treatment for the care recipient (Mullan, 1993; Mockus Parks and Novielli, 2000), and negative tension in relations (Biegel et al., 1993); and b) other authors have found ambiguous results, concluding that respite care has a varied impact on the carer burden (Lawton, Brody and Saperstein, 1989; Forde and Pearlman, 1999). It has even been stated that the home help service is important for carers but that its role is not so great as to be able to reduce the stress felt by carers in the provision of care (Decima Research Inc. and Health Canada, 2002; Carretero, Garcés and Ródenas, in press).

Also, while the use of a day centre offers the carer a real reduction in the care burden and an improvement in self-perceived health as a result of a regular daily rest from care of the dependant (Tárraga et al., 2000), this effect has been seen to disappear when the carer gets used to receiving this type of support, with the carer then reverting to a higher perception of the care burden (Jones, 1992).

In another case, when comparing carers that use respite services with others who do not, for a period in excess of three months, there is a significant decrease in the care burden. However, the primary stressors tied to the role of carer such as role captivity and concern about various aspects of carer engagement did not change at all (Zarit, 1996).

The available results which place doubt on the effectiveness of formal assistance as a mediator in the care stress process suggest that there are a number of factors that may affect either the resource itself or the carer, without resulting in the expected positive effects on the carer burden. These aspects are reviewed below.

Firstly, the use for formal support may have adverse effects if the care offered is not reliable, good-quality or does not meet the needs of both carer and care recipient are (Kahana, Biegel and Wylde, 1994; Bass, 2002). Hawranik and Strain (2000) found that the carers of elderly parents using home help felt a greater burden. The authors explain that these results might be because the demands for care from dependent parents were so great that, even if formal services were used, the burden did not decrease.

Secondly, formal services were often found to be under-used (Mullan, 1993; Zarit, 1996), with carers using minimal formal care services so receiving little relief (Aneshensel et al., 1995).

Another explanation for the contradictory results found regarding the usefulness of respite services for reducing the care burden is that informal carers request such resources when they are already at crisis stage, when the burden is excessive (Rodríguez, 1999). Carers wait too long before resorting to a respite service and ask for it when the dependent person is already at an advanced stage of the illness (Knight, Lutzky y Macofsky - Urban, 1993; Zarit, 1996). In fact, after reviewing several studies on the impact of the use of respite services on carer burden, Knight and co-workers (Knight, Lutzky y Macofsky – Urban, 1993) found only a moderate effect of respite services on alleviation of the care burden. For this reason, it has been suggested that better results can be obtained for the carer burden when the respite service is used in a preventive way. This means that the formal resource would prevent the carer's collapse instead of being an emergency measure used once the carer has become totally exhausted (International Psychogeriatric Association, 2002). It has been shown that early intervention results in greater alleviation of carer stress and other negative consequences of care-giving (Lyons and Zarit, 1999).

There are several possible reasons why carers put off the search for formal aid. For example, it has been seen that carers think they will be able to provide all the care themselves (Zarit, 1996) and are concerned about the quality and reliability of the formal service (Zarit, MaloneBeach and Spore, 1988; Noelker and Bass, 1989) or about the long-term cost of the service which might prevent the institutionalisation of the dependent person when the need arises (Zarit, 1996). On this last consideration, carers would prefer to save in order to have funds available when care is no longer an option. Finally, some carers reject the possibility of receiving formal aid from the respite services (Gottlieb and Johnson, 2000).

Other explanations for the disparity of results of the effect of respite services on carer burden is that such resources provide insufficient relief for carers (Berry, Zarit and Rabatin, 1991; Jarrot and Zarit, 1995). On the one hand, the respite services do not give the carer sufficient time to take time off from caring (Berry, Zarit and Rabatin, 1991; Zarit, 1996; Carretero, Garcés and Ródenas, 2006). Carers feel a substantial level of stress which they are relatively resistant to change so, if just a few hours of respite are offered, there is unlikely to be much of an effect on the carer burden (Zarit, 1996). On the other hand, carers use the respite time to deal with other tasks for other family members (Berry, Zarit and Rabatin, 1991). Zarit (1994) states that it is wrong to expect carers to rest or undertake pleasurable activities during respite time to recover their psychological resources.

It has also been noted that the contradictory results on the effectiveness of respite services for carers may be due to the fact that no prior evaluation of the carer is carried out. In order to devise intervention with informal carers, prior evaluation should first determine the objectives of the programme before determining what results can be expected and what measurement tools are needed (Friss, 2002). It has been stated that it is essential to understand the carer's role, the many stressors involved and the particular situation of the family carer for the design of any care plan (Gaugler, Kane and Langlois, 2000; Friss, 2002).

4.2. Psycho-Social Programmes

Another important type of intervention that has been seen to be effective for alleviating the carer burden, in addition to respite programmes, are *psycho-social or psycho-educational programmes* (Zarit, 1990b). This type of intervention is designed in a general way to improve or increase the carer's skills for dealing with care situations (Zarit, 1990b). The general objectives are, on the one hand, to reduce the burden, stress and distress felt by carers and, on the other, to improve the quality of care received by the dependent persons (Montorio, Díaz e Izal, 1995).

These programmes use a varied range of intervention procedures, strategies and formats: support groups, self-care and mutual care, training in cognitive-behavioural techniques such as problem solving, stress management, etc. As explained below, they are mostly based on information, learning skills and emotional support. It could be said that this type of intervention includes the learning of strategies for coping with the specific circumstances of the care situation as well as social support in the form of assistance from the informal support network (Zarit, 1990b; Yanguas and Pérez, 1997).

Some programmes have been drawn up that bring together different elements of intervention (Brodaty, 1992; International Psychogeriatric Association, 2002), that is:

a) Psychological intervention, including emotional ventilation, the feeling of belonging to a group, training and mutual support, counselling, cognitive therapy, training in relaxation and learning to manage stress, self-care, communication and interpersonal relations.
b) Educational intervention focusing on the provision of information, improving skills in home care, the development of therapeutic skills, problem solving, behavioural techniques, planning of urgent financial and legal matters. Research has shown that it is very important that the family or a family member is trained in skills for solving problems relating to the dependent family member (Houts et al., 1996).

Studies on the effectiveness of psycho-social intervention and on different techniques are still rare if compared with research on the consequences of informal care (Zarit and Leitsch, 2001). Support groups have traditionally been one of the main exponents for this type of programme (Zarit, 1990b) and much research has been carried out on them and on other similar psycho-social interventions to reduce the burden (Mockus Parks and Novielli, 2000). In general, there are studies that confirm the positive results of such programmes (Sánchez, Mouronte and Olazarán, 2001; Gallagher-Thomspon et al., 2003) as well as others indicating that their effects are limited (Zarit, 1990b; Knight, Lutzky and Macofsky - Urban, 1993; Sörensen, Pinquart and Duberstein, 2002).

In general, the use of different psycho-social components has differential effects on the burden and mental health indicators (Losada et al., 2004). Research has found, for example, that counselling and support groups, in combination with respite services, have direct, positive effects on the adoption of healthy conduct (Gallart and Connell, 1998) and help carers to maintain their role as carers for longer, with less stress and greater satisfaction (Mittleman et al., 1996). Mittleman and co-workers (1996) found that the combination of intervention including group and individual counselling sessions as well as obligatory participation in support groups delayed the need for institutionalising the dependent person by an average of 329 days.

In samples of carers of persons suffering from dementia, the research has focused especially on the potential effectiveness of educational components, given that the conduct of carers towards the demented person has a direct, significant impact on the patients. The efficiency of such strategies may be based on the fact that the carer's reaction to the dependant's symptoms may be as great in the development of the burden as the pathology of the care recipient. Sometimes, the conduct of carers of demented persons – such as making sudden, unexpected changes to the patient's routine and environment or being excessively critical – may actually aggravate the psychological and behavioural symptoms of the disease, which are very closely related to the carer burden. Such conduct arises because many carers believe that the psychological and behavioural symptoms of the dementia are under the control of the patient, interpreting their forgetfulness as irresponsibility, their irascibility as lack of fondness, their repetitive questioning as deliberate obstructiveness. These reactions increase the likelihood that they will express criticism or hostility towards the patient, while generating emotional distress in themselves. Interventions on carer conduct when interacting with the patient may lengthen the carer's capacity for providing care at home and guarantee quality of life for both parties (International Psychogeriatric Association, 2002).

An example can be seen in the studies carried out by Niederehe and co-workers (Niederehe et al., 1983; Niederehe and Funk, 1987) who showed the impact of behavioural interaction between the carer and the care recipient. Their results showed that carers who used authoritarian or evasive answers in their interaction with the patient felt a greater burden and greater psychological distress than those whose answers supported and encouraged the dependent person.

Haley (1997) showed that educational support was more beneficial for carers when it focused on modifying conduct. Other studies, however, have pinpointed the inefficiency of this type of programme on the subjective burden (Demers and Lavoie, 1996; Losada et al., 2004) and the depression symptoms of the carer (Zarit, Zarit y Reever, 1982) and stress the importance of cognitive intervention to correct the irrational thoughts that are associated with care (Losada et al., 2004). For example, Losada and co-workers (2004) compared a group of carers of family members suffering from dementia which received a programme of cognitive/behavioural intervention to modify their dysfunctional thinking on care with another group which received training on problem solving to modify the patient's behavioural problems. The two groups were compared with a control group. The authors of this research found that, after the intervention, the carers who underwent the cognitive/behavioural programme reported less perceived stress, fewer behavioural problems in their family members and fewer irrational thoughts than the other two groups. It has been argued that this result could be due to the fact that the behavioural changes adopted to change the behaviour of the patient with dementia might lead to a degree of distress in the carer (Fiore et al., 1983), in that they might be more aware of the limitation of the care recipient (Zarit, Zarit and Reever, 1982) or because they have an indirect effect on the burden (Zarit, 1990b).

Certain limitations have also been found in psycho-social programmes which might reduce their effectiveness on the carer burden. Firstly, it has been pointed out that psycho-social programmes address the carer alone, and cover neither the care recipient nor the interaction between them both. Such interventions are designed to limit, diminish and control the negative consequences of care for the carer and to reduce certain behaviour that can be modified in dependent persons and that aggravates the carer burden. But they do not take into account the wishes and values of the dependent person (Yanguas and Pérez, 1997).

Secondly, programmes for intervention offer too much content to the extent that the maximum time recommended by some authors for intervention with carers – 8 to 10 sessions (Gallagher –Thomspon et al., 2000) - prevents thorough training in all the skills covered by the programme. Moreover, the instruments used to prove the effectiveness of interventions usually measure the overall burden or stress. It is known, however, that the carer burden process is multi-dimensional, and that brief intervention cannot work changes in every one of these dimensions (Zarit, 1990b).

Finally, a large number of carers refuse to participate in programmes designed to reduce their psychological distress (Losada et al., 2004), either because they do not consider they need help (Caserta et al., 1987) or because they do not have time to attend the intervention sessions (Gallagher –Thomspon et al., 2000).

5. Conclusion: The Best Solution for the Future

After this extensive review of the programmes used in research to relieve the carer burden, we can conclude that the two types of programmes are very useful in helping carers to cope with the stress of the caring situation. However, there are a number of limitations which means that the role of formal social support as regards the care burden is not yet clear, so further research is needed.

In this sense, recent research has proposed the suitability of combining both types of programs—the respite services and psycho-educational programs—to deal with the excessive burden placed on informal caregivers by dependent people (Carretero et al., 2007, 2008; Garcés et al., 2008). These interventions would thus be able to reduce the burden for informal carers and their emotional distress, increase their well-being and quality of life and postpone burnout. These benefits are noted in the literature (Brubacker, 1990; Friss et al., 1995).

Regarding this, our research indicates that the use of In-Home Help Service seems to be an optimal respite option to combined with psychosocial support, as it is an important social resource which usually is available in all the Social Service Systems, which would be useful to provide respite to the caregivers of dependent people for their care tasks, at the same time, it has been recognised as a suitable formula for addressing the problem of delivering long-term care to dependent people (Council of Europe, 1998). Its use entails a reduction in care costs (Garcés, 2000), and home-based care is preferred by dependent people and also delays and prevents institutionalization, while promoting well-being, longevity and quality of life (Havens, 1999; John, Hennessy, Dyeson and Garrett, 2001; OECD, 2005).

Concretely, our data and the revised research suggest that the mental health of the informal carer can be improved through an In-Home Help Service with diversified services in the support of daily life activities of dependent people, with an appropriate duration of them according to their needs, in order to allow the caregiver to rest in a sufficient way and decrease his/her excessive burden levels.

This service needs to be combined with a psycho-educational program to alleviate the emotional discomfort of the informal caregivers and provide them with skills and strategies to face the challenge of caregiving. Concretely, we refer to psychological support by means of techniques such as ventilation of emotions, cognitive therapy, training in relaxation, etc., in order to relieve the emotional discomfort and the heavy burden as well as give educational support, above all focused on the incorporation of cognitive–behavioral techniques to modify the irrational thoughts of the caregivers—for example, "I must not request help from my family relatives, since they have their own lives and problems"—or of behavioral techniques in order to know how to request help. It must inform and train the informal caregivers about the dependency and physical decay by means of teaching coping strategies such as the redefinition of the disease or to accept the dependency as a process associated with aging or with the disease of the patient; and training in skills for the assistance and care directed to senior citizens and to those with a low education level, which increases their perception of competence in the care of a dependent senior citizen and thus prevents the abandonment of the care. In general, these specific psychosocial components have already demonstrated their effectiveness on the informal caregivers' burden in oncological patients and those with insanity (Gallagher-Thompson et al., 2003; Haley, 2003; Patterson et al., 2000; Zarit and Leitsch, 2001). The psychological and educational support must be included in the In-Home Help Services to increase their effectiveness in the relief of the burden as other authors in more specific fields have established, such as the informal caregivers of patients with dementia or hemodialysis (Belasco and Sesso, 2002; Brodaty, 1992; Galltart and Connell, 1997). As noted by Pinquart and Sörensen (2006), special care should be given to the quality of these psychoeducational programs, particularly in terms of more structuring and intensity of the interventions.

It is especially important to focus this type of program on the female population, insofar as recent data indicates that in around 80% of the cases in Europe, the informal care of dependent senior citizens is assumed by a woman (EUROFAMCARE, 2006).

Finally, continuing in the study of other variables of the dependent person and the care context associated to the caregiver burden, in order to analyze the characteristics that can be modifiable in psycho-educational interventions is needed. Financial support from the governments for the research in this field is fundamental to reach this objective (Carretero et al.,2007; Carretero et al., 2006).

Acknowledgments

Acknowledgments to the Ministry of Science and Education (SEC 2002 - 02634) and the Consellerías de Sanitat y de Bienestar Social of the Generalitat Valenciana (Spain).

References

Aneshensel C, Pearlin L, Mullan J, Zarit SH, Whitlatch CJ. 1995. *Profiles in caregiving: The unexpected career*. Academic Press: New York.

Bains M. 2003. Projecting future needs: Long-term projections of public expenditure on health and long-term care for EU Member States. In: A Disease-based Comparison of Health Systems: What is best and at what cost? OECD. OECD: Paris; 145-162.

Bass DM. 2002. Content and implementation of a caregiver assessment. Issue Brief, National Family Caregiver Support Program. U.S. Administration on Aging: Washington, DC.

Biegel D, Schulz R. 1998. Caregiving and caregiver interventions in aging and mental illness. *Fam Relat* 48: 345-354.

Bourgeois M, Schulz R, Burgio L. 1996. Interventions for caregivers of patients with Alzheimer's disease: A review and analysis of content, process, and outcomes. *Int J Aging Hum Dev* 43: 35-92.

Brodaty, H. and Hadzi-Pavlovic, D. (1990). Psychosocial effects on carers of living with persons with dementia. *Australian New Zealand Journal of Psychiatry*, 24, 351–361.

Carretero, S. et al. (2008). The informal caregiver's burden of dependent people: Theory and empirical review, *Arch Gerontol Geriatr*, doi:10.1016/j.archger.2008.05.004

Carretero, S., Garcés, J., Ródenas, F., 2007. Evaluation of the home help service and its impact on the informal caregiver's burden of dependent elders. *Int. J. Geriatr. Psych.* 22, 738-749.

Carretero, S.; Garcés, J. and Ródenas, F. and Sanjosé, V. (2006). La Sobrecarga de las Cuidadoras de Personas Dependientes. Valencia: Tirant Lo Blanc.

Council of Europe. 1998. Recommendation No. R (98) 9 of the Committee of Ministers to Member States on Dependence (Adopted by the Committee of Ministers on 18 September 1998 at the 641st meeting of the Ministers'Deputies).

Decima Research Inc, Health Canada. 2002. National Profile of Family Caregivers in Canada – 2002. Final Report. Health Canada: Ottawa.

Deimling, G. and Bass, D. (1986). Symptoms of Mental Impairment among Elderly Adults and Their Effects on Family Caregivers. *Journal of Gerontology*, 41, 778–784.

Dunkin, J.J. and Anderson – Hanley, C. (1998). Dementia caregiver burden: a review of the literature and guidelines for assessment and intervention. *Neurology, 51 (suppl. 1),* S53 – S60.

Eurostat. 1999. European Community Household Panel. European Community: Bruxelles.

Family Caregiver Alliance (2001). *Fact Sheet: Selected Caregiver Statistics.* San Francisco, CA: Family Caregiver Alliance.

Forde OT, Pearlman S. 1999. Breakaway: A social supplement to caregivers' support groups. *Am J Alz Dis* 14: 120-124.

Friss, L. (2002). The *State of the Art: Caregiver assessment in practice settings.* San Francisco: Family Caregiver Alliance, National Center on Caregiving.

Gallagher-Thompson, D.; Coon, D.W.; Solano, N.; Ambler, C.; Rabinowitz, Y. and Thompson, L.W. (2003). Change in indices of distress among Latino and Anglo female caregivers of elderly relatives with dementia: site-specific results from the REACH national collaborative study. *Gerontologist, 43*(4), 580-591.

Gallagher-Thompson, D.; Coon, D.W.; Solano, N.; Ambler, C.; Rabinowitz, Y. and Thompson, L.W. (2003). Change in indices of distress among Latino and Anglo female caregivers of elderly relatives with dementia: site-specific results from the REACH national collaborative study. *Gerontologist*, 43(4), 580-591.

Gallagher-Thompson, D.; Lovett, S.; Rose, J.; McKibbin, C.; Coon, D.; Futterman, A. and Thompson, L. (2000). Impact of psychoeducational interventions on distressed family caregivers. *Journal of Clinical Geropsychology*, *6*, 91-110.

Garcés J, Ródenas F, Sanjosé V. 2003. Towards a new welfare state: the social sustainability principle and health care strategies. *Health Policy* 65: 201-215.

Garcés J, Ródenas F, Sanjosé V. 2004. Care needs among the dependent population in Spain: an empirical approach. *Health Soc Care Community* 12: 466-474.

Garcés J. 2000. La nueva sostenibilidad social. Ariel: Barcelona.

Garcés, J. et al. (2008). Variables related to the informal caregivers' burden of dependent senior citizens in Spain, *Arch Gerontol Geriatr*,doi:10.1016/j.archger.2008.03.004

Gaugler JE, Kane RA, Langlois J. 2000. Assessment of Family Caregivers of Older Adults. In *Assessing Older Persons: Measures, Meaning and Practical Applications*, Kane RL, Kane RA (eds). Oxford University Press: New York; 320–359.

George, L.E. and Gwyther, L.P. (1986). Caregiver Well-Being: A Multidimensional Examination of Family Caregivers of Demented Adults. *Gerontologist, 26*, 253–259.

Grad, J. and Sainsbury, P. (1963). Mental Illness and the Family. *The Lancet*, 1, 544–547.

Grundy E, Glaser K. 2000. Sociodemographic differences in the onset and progression of disability in early old age: a longitudinal study. *Age Ageing* 29: 149-157.

Grunfeld, E.; Coyle, D.; Whelan, T.; Clinch, J.; Reyno, L.; Earle, C.C.; Willan, A.; Viola, R.; Coristine, M.; Janz, T. and Glossop, R. (2004). Family caregiver burden: results of a longitudinal study of breast cancer patients and their principal caregivers. *Canadian Medical Association Journal,* 170 (12), 1795-1801.

Havens B. 1999. Home-based and long-term care. World Health Organization: Geneva.

Havens, B. (1999). *Home-based and long-term care*. Geneva: World Health Organization.

Hawranik PG, Strain LA. 2000. Health of Informal Caregivers: Effects of gender, employment, and use of home care services. University of Manitoba, Centre on Aging: Winnipeg (Manitoba).

IMSERSO (2004*). Situación y evolución del apoyo informal a los mayores en España. Avance de resultados: informe descriptivo*. Madrid: Ministerio de Trabajo y Asuntos Sociales, Secretaría General de Asuntos Sociales, IMSERSO.

INE (2004). *Panel de Hogares de la Unión Europea 1994-1999*. www.ine.es.

International Psychogeriatric Association (IPA) (2002). Behavioral and Psychological Symptoms of Dementia (BPSD) Educational Pack. International Psychogeriatric Association.

EUROFAMCARE (2006). Services for supporting family carers of elderly people in Europe: characteristics, coverage and usage (summary of main findings from EUROFAMCARE). Available at http://www.uke.de/extern/eurofamcare/documents/deliverables/summary_of_findings.pdf

Jacobzone S. 1999. Ageing and care for frail elderly persons: an overview of international perspectives - Occasional Papers nº 38. Paris: OECD, Directorate for Education, Employment, Labour and Social Affairs, Labour Market and Social Policy.

Jarrot, S.E. and Zarit, S.H. (1995). *The effects of day care on time usage by employed and non-employed caregivers*. 48th Annual Scientific Meeting of the Gerontological Society of America Council.

Jenson, J. and Jacobzone, S. (2000). Care allowances for the frail elderly and their impact on women care-givers. Labour Market and Social Policy – Occasional Papers nº 41. Paris: OECD; Directorate for Education, Employment, Labour and Social Affairs; Employment, Labour and Social Affairs Committee.

John R, Hennessy CH, Dyeson TB, Garrett MD. 2001. Toward the conceptualization and measurement of caregiver burden among Pueblo Indian family caregivers. *Gerontologist* 41: 210–219.

Jones GMM. 1992. A communication model of dementia: with particular reference to Alzheimer´s disease. In Caregiving in dementia, Jones GMM, Miesen BML (eds). Routledge: London; 437-453

Kahana E, Biegel D, Wykle M (ed.). 1994. *Family caregiving across the lifespan*. Sage Publications: Newbury Park, CA.

Knight, B. G., Lutzky, S. M. and Macofsky-Urban, F. (1993). A meta-analytic review of interventions for caregiver distress: Recommendations for future research. *The Gerontologist*, 3, 240-248.

Knight, B. G., Lutzky, S. M. and Macofsky-Urban, F. (1993). A meta-analytic review of interventions for caregiver distress: Recommendations for future research. *The Gerontologist*, 3, 240-248.

Lawton M, Brody E, Saperstein A. 1989. A controlled study of respite service for caregivers of Alzheimer's patients. Gerontologist 29: 8 – 16.

Lazarus, R.S. and Folkman, S. (1984). *Stress, Appraisal and Coping*. New York: Springer.

Lee SL, Colditz GA, Berkman LF, Kawachi I. 2003. Caregiving and risk of coronary heart disease in U.S. women: A prospective study. *Am J Prev Med* 24: 113–119.

Logdon RG, Gibbons LE, McCurry SM, Teri L. 1999. Quality of life in Alzheimer's disease: patient and caregiver reports. *Gerontologist* 5: 21 – 32.

Lyons, K.S. and Zarit, S.H. (1999). Formal and Informal Support: The great divide. International *Journal of Geriatric Psychiatry, 14,* 183 – 196.

Mahoney FI, Barthel DW. 1965. Functional Evaluation: The Barthel Index. *Md State Med J* 14: 61-65.

MaloneBeach EE, Zarit SH, Spore DL. 1992. Caregivers' perceptions of case management and community-based services: Barriers to service use. *J Appl Gerontol* 11: 146-159.

Malonebeach, E. and Zarit, S. (1995). Dimensions of social support and social conflict as predictors of caregiver depression. *International Psychogeriatrics*, 7 (1), 25-36.

Marks, N.; Lambert, J. D. and Choi, H. (2002). Transitions to caregiving, gender, and psychological well-being: A prospective U.S. national study. *Journal of Marriage and Family*, 64, 657–667.

Martín M, Salvadó I, Nadal S, Miji LC, Rico JM, Lanz P, Taussig MI. 1996. Adaptación para nuestro medio de la Escala de Sobrecarga del Cuidador (Caregiver Burden Interview) de Zarit. *Rev Esp Geriatr Gerontol* 6: 338-346.

McGuire, P. y Fulmer, T. (1997). Elder abuse. In *Geriatric medicine* (3rd ed.), Cassel CK, Cohen HJ, Larson EB, Meier DE, Resnick NM, Rubenstein LZ, Sorenson LB (eds). Springer-Verlag: New York; 855-864.

Mears, J. (1998). *Paying for Care: Repercussions for Women Who Care, the case of Australia*. University of Western Sydney, Department of Social Policy and Human Services, Faculty of Arts and Social Sciences: Mimeo.

Mockus Parks S, Novielli KD. 2000. A practical guide to caring for caregivers. *Am Fam Physician* 15: 2215 – 2219.

Montgomery, R. (1989). As AARP grows, so does criticism of its priorities. *Seattle Times*, 12.

Montgomery, R.J.V. and Borgatta, E.F. (1989). The Effect of Alternative Support Strategies on Family Caregivers. *The Gerontologist, 29*, 457–464.

Montgomery, R.J.V.; Gonyea, J.G. and Hooyman, N.R. (1985). Caregiving and the experience of subjective burden. *Family Relations, 34*, 19–26.

Montorio I, Izal M, López A, Sánchez M. 1998. La Entrevista de Carga del Cuidador. Utilidad y validez del concepto de carga. *Anales de Psicología* 14: 229-248.

Mullan JT. 1993. Barriers to the use of formal services among Alzheimer's caregivers. In *Caregiving systems: Informal and formal helpers*, Zarit SH, Pearlin LI, Schaie KW (eds). Erlbaum: Hillsdale NJ; 241 – 259.

National Alliance for Caregiving, AARP. 1997. Family caregiving in the U.S.: Findings from a national survey. National Alliance for Caregiving y AARP: Washington, DC.

Navaie-Waliser, M. Spriggs, A. and Feldman, P.H. (2002). Informal caregiving. Differential experiences by gender. *Medical Care, 40*, 1249-1259.

Noonan, A.E. and Tennstedt, S.L. (1997). Meaning in caregiving and its contribution to caregiver well-being. *Gerontologist*, 37, 785-94.

OECD. 1998. The Future of Female-Dominated Occupations. OECD: Paris.

OECD. 2005. The OECD Health Project : Long – term care for older people. OECD: Paris.

Pacolet J, Bouten R, Lanoye H, Versieck K. 2000. Social Protection for Dependency in Old Age: A study of the fifteen EU Member States and Norway. Ashgate: Hampshire.

Pearlin LI, Mullan JT, Semple SJ, Skaff MM. 1990. Caregiving and the Stress Process: An Overview of Concepts and Their Measures. *Gerontologist* 30: 583–594.

Pearlin LI, Turner HA, Semple SJ. 1989. Coping and the mediation of caregiver stress. In Alzheimer's disease treatment and family stress: Directions for research, Light E, Lebowitz B (eds). U.S. Government Printing Office: Washington, DC; 198 – 217.

Pearlin, L.I. and Skaff, M.M. (1995). Stressors in adaptation in late life. E M. Gatz (ed.): *Emerging issues in mental health and aging*. Washington: APA.

Pearlin, L.I.; Mullan, J.T.; Semple, S.J. and Skaff, M.M. (1990). Caregiving and the Stress Process: An Overview of Concepts and Their Measures. *Gerontologist,* 30, 583–594.

Pearlin, L.I.; Turner, H.A. and Semple, S.J. (1989). Coping and the mediation of caregiver stress. En E. Light and B. Lebowitz (eds): *Alzheimer's disease treatment and family stress: Directions for research*. Washington, DC: U.S. Government Printing Office, pp. 198 – 217.

Pinquart, M. and Sörensen. S. (2006). Helping caregivers of persons with dementia: which interventions work and how large are their effects? *International Psychogeriatrics*, 18:4, 577 – 595.

Semple, S.J. (1992). Conflict in Alzheimer's carefiving families: Its dimensions and consequences. *Gerontologist, 32*, 648 – 655.

Vevren, L. (2006). Advancing International Long-Term Care Initiatives through Cross-Atlantic Exchange. In *Global Report on Aging, Special Issue* 2006. AARP.

Wackerbarth S. 1998. A predictive model of nursing home placement: the perspective of caregivers with Alzheimer's disease. AHSR and FHSR Annual Meeting Abstract Book 13: 195 – 196.

Yee JL, Schulz R. 2000. Gender Differences in Psychiatric Morbidity Among Family Caregivers: A Review and Analysis. *Gerontologist* 2: 147-164.

Zarit (1989). Issues and directions in Family intervention research. En E. Light and B.D. Lebowitz (eds): *Alzheimer, and Family Stress: Directions for research.* Washington, D.C.: US Government Printing Office, 458 – 486.

Zarit SH, Gaugler JE, Jarrot SE. 1999. Useful services for families: Research findings and directions. *Int J Geriatr Psych* 14: 165 – 181.

Zarit SH, Orr NK, Zarit JM. 1985. *The hidden victims of Alzheimer's disease. Families under stress*. New York University Press: Nueva York.

Zarit SH, Reever KE, Bach-Peterson J. 1980. Relatives of the impaired elderly: correlates of feelings of burden. *Gerontologist* 20: 649-654.

Zarit SH, Zarit JM. 1983. *The Memory and behavior problems checklist.* University Park: Pennsylvania State University.

Zarit SH. 1998. Dementia: caregivers and stress. Community paper series: paper 8. Centre on Aging, University of Victoria: Victoria, BC.

Zarit SH. 2002. Caregiver's Burden. In Family and professional carers: findings lead to action, Andrieu S, Aquino JP. Serdi Edition y Fondation Médéric Alzheimer: Paris; 20-24

Zarit, S.H. (1990). Interventions with Frail Elders and Their Families: Are They Effective and Why?. En M.A. Parris Stephens, J.H. Crowther, S.E. Hobfoll and D.L. Tennenbaum (eds): *Stress and Coping in Later Life Families*. New York: Hemisphere Publishing Company.

Zarit, S.H. (1990). Interventions with Frail Elders and Their Families: Are They Effective and Why?. En M.A. Parris Stephens, J.H. Crowther, S.E. Hobfoll and D.L. Tennenbaum (eds): *Stress and Coping in Later Life Families*. New York: Hemisphere Publishing Company.

Zarit, S.H. (1996). *Families at the Crossroads: Caring for Disabled Older People.* Pennsylvania: Penn Sate University, Gerontology Center, College of Health and Human Development.

Zarit, S.H. (1996). Families at the Crossroads: Caring for Disabled Older People. Pennsylvania: Penn Sate University, Gerontology Center, College of Health and Human Development.

Zarit, S.H. (2002). Caregiver's Burden. In S. Andrieu and J.P. Aquino: *Family and professional carers: findings lead to action.* Paris: Serdi Edition and Fondation Médéric Alzheimer.

Zarit, S.H.; Reever, K.E. and Bach-Peterson, J. (1980). Relatives of the impaired elderly: correlates of feelings of burden. *Gerontologist, 20*, 649-654.

In: Psychiatric Research Trends: Dreams and Geriatric Psychiatry ISBN 978-1-60741-760-6
Editors: Daniella M. Montez, pp.47-66

Chapter 3

A Review of the Outcome of Delirium in Elderly Patients

Dimitrios Adamis*,1 and Alastair J. D. Macdonald†,2
[1]Research and Academic Institute of Athens, Greece,
Department of Ageing and Health, Guy's and St. Thomas' NHS Foundation Trust, London, UK
[2]Institute of Psychiatry, London, UK, HSPR Department, London, UK

Abstract

Introduction: Delirium is a neuropsychiatric syndrome defined by acute onset, fluctuating course and disturbances of consciousness, attention, orientation, memory, thought, perception and behavior. The course of delirium has often been described as transient, in which recovery is likely to be complete if the underlying etiological factor is cured. Older people, who have delirium, experience a range of poor clinical outcomes including significant increases in cognitive impairment, functional disability, increased length of hospital stay, psychological distress, high rates of institutionalization, and high rates of death, independent of many socio-demographic and clinical variables.

Methods: Databases were searched with the keywords 'delirium' or 'acute confusion' and 'outcome'. The keywords 'cognitive impairment,' 'functional disability', 'length of hospital stay', 'mortality', 'institutionalization', 'psychological stress' have also been used in combination with the former. Studies have been categorized in relation to six outcomes: a) mortality, b) cognitive impairment, c) functional decline, d) length of hospital stay, e) discharge destination, and f) psychological morbidity.

Results: There are methodological problems and heterogeneity in the examined studies. Regarding cognitive impairment the examined studies suggest that delirium is associated with an increased risk of subsequent cognitive decline. Not all studies have

---

* Corresponding author: Dr. Dimitrios Adamis MSc, GradStat, MD Consultant in Old Age Psychiatry, Research and Academic Institute of Athens, Greece, 27 Themistokleous Street and Akadimias, Athens, 106 77, Greece, Tel/Fax:+30 210 33 040 43, email: dimaadamis@yahoo.com.

† Professor of Old Age Psychiatry, Institute of Psychiatry, London, UK Room HO.09, HSPR Department, David Goldberg Building, de Crespigny Park, London SE5 8AP Tel +44 203 228 7735, email alastair.macdonald@iop.kcl.ac.uk

found an association of delirium with subsequent functional impairment. Similarly there are conflicting results among studies which examined length of stay. Most studies agree that there is a relationship between delirium and mortality and especially for those with pre-existing dementia. A majority of studies have found that delirium is associated with a high rate of institutional care. A small number of studies have examined the psychological stress that delirium cause patients and also relatives and nurses.

Discussion: Studies generally agree that there is an association of delirium and subsequent cognitive decline and institutionalization. There is no conclusive evidence about the relationship between delirium and functional disability, length of stay or mortality. Given that there is an association between functional decline and cognitive decline, delirium may induce a long term or even permanent cognitive decline which then manifests as functional decline. The contribution of delirium to mortality is complex. Perhaps underling pathophysiological mechanisms common to both delirium and dementia are related to mortality. It is not yet certain that delirium prolongs hospital stay once other confounding factors are controlled for. The notion of subsyndromal delirium is briefly discussed.

Conclusions: There are many methodological and ethical concerns which obstruct delirium research. It is clear from this review that delirium has very serious adverse outcomes and it is necessary to develop biological markers which can allow a focus of preventative measures on those at most risk of developing it.

INTRODUCTION

Definitions

Delirium is a common neuropsychiatric disorder in elderly hospitalized patients; a condition that is often presented in medical, surgical, intensive care units (ICU) and in other acute, sub-acute or rehabilitation settings. It is known by various names, including organic brain syndrome, acute brain failure, acute organic reaction, ICU psychosis, encephalopathy, acute confusion or acute confusional state. Lindesay et al. (1990). Although some of these names still are in use, the two current classification systems (DSM-IV and ICD-10) both adopt the word delirium in their definition. According to ICD-10 delirium is defined as an etiologically non specific organic cerebral syndrome with concurrent disturbances of consciousness, perception, thinking and cognition, psychomotor manifestations, and disturbances of the sleep-wake schedule. (Cooper and WHO, 1994).

Similar definition has been given by APA (1994) in DSM-IV where delirium is defined as a disorder of acute onset, over hours to days, followed by a course of fluctuation in the level of consciousness, attention and cognition, sometimes accompanied by delusions or hallucinations. Whilst the use of those two international classifications (ICD, DSM) can increase the concurred validity of a diagnosis between professionals, and facilitate communication between them, there are criticisms that have led to the new notion of subsyndromal delirium.

Schmidt et al. (2004) argue that the dichotomous nature of diagnosis is arbitrary especially when certain forms of psychopathology are best viewed as dimensional phenomena. Such dimensional symptoms in delirium might include psychomotor activity, consciousness, attention, speech disturbances and, in inpatients, the sleep-wake cycle. Indeed, investigators have commented on the weakness of a categorical approach to the diagnosis of delirium. Levkoff et al. (1996) in their seminal work suggested that delirium represents a spectrum of neurobehavioral impairment and they used the term "Subsyndromal Delirium" (SSD) to describe those who did not meet the full criteria of delirium but who had some delirium symptoms. Patients with SSD fall on a continuum between those with DSM-defined delirium and those with no symptoms of delirium. Levkoff et al. (2004) reviewed published studies to examine whether findings supported the notion of delirium as a spectrum disorder or whether SSD represented a categorically separate diagnosis from delirium as defined by the DSM. They concluded that SSD may be the either the prodrome for full DSM-defined delirium or may have adverse outcomes of its own - intermediate between those of no delirium and the full syndrome.

Epidemiology of Delirium

Most studies considering the prevalence and incident rates of delirium in elderly populations have been carried out in medical and surgical inpatients. However the estimated prevalence and incidence rates vary between studies, perhaps this is due to conceptual and methodological issues. (Lindesay et al. 2002).

A number of earlier studies which involved medical inpatients showed a high rate of prevalent delirium. Flint and Richard (1956) estimated a prevalence rate of 49% while Bedford (1959) reported a very high prevalence rate of 80%. Simon and Caham (1963) reported a lower prevalence rate of 13% but they excluded all patients with dementia.

Intermediate rates of 25% have been reported by Hodkinson (1973) using a diagnostic method of distinguishing delirium from dementia by the course of the illness alone. More recent studies (e.g. Cole et al. 2002, Laurila et al. 2004, Naughton et al. 2005, Korevaar et al. 2005) reported a range between 13% and 40.9%. The criteria used were DSM-IIIR and DSM-IV.

Regarding incidence rates- usually defined as per admission- earlier studies reported a range of 10% (Bleuler et al. 1966) to 53% (Chisholm et al. 1982), while more recent large studies on elderly medical inpatients (e.g. Villalpando-Berumen et al. 2003 and Bourdel-Marchasson et al. 2004) found an incidence rate of delirium of between 4% and 12%.

Although the estimation of prevalence and incidence rates are not consistent among published studies, both over the years but also between settings, it seems that delirium is very common in elderly inpatients; more than 20% of over 70 year- old patients are likely to be delirious on admission, while more than 10% develop delirium subsequently, most within the first few days (Inouye et al. 1993), and even higher in patients with cancer, terminal illness or in ICU (Leentjens et al. 2008, Pandharipande et al. 2008)

Delirium is not always a recoverable condition in elderly medical inpatients (Levkoff et al. 1992, Rudberg et al. 1997), and has been associated with important adverse outcomes, including mortality, persistent cognitive impairment, functional decline, increased hospital stay, placement in care homes and psychological morbidity in the survivors.

In this chapter previous studies related to these outcomes will be reviewed, including factors that may contribute to outcomes, and a discussion will follow in which the use of the outcome as a critical factor in the definition of delirium will be presented.

Method

The database MEDLINE, EMBASE, PsycINFO, SCOPUS, all EBM Reviews (OVID) were searched using the keywords 'delirium', 'acute confusion', 'acute confusional state', and 'outcome'. Also the keywords 'cognitive impairment', 'functional disability', 'length of hospital stay', 'mortality', 'institutionalization', 'mental recall', 'psychological stress', 'affect', 'outcome' were used each in combination with the former. Studies were categorized in relation to six outcomes: a) mortality, b) cognitive impairment, c) functional decline, d) length of hospital stay, e) discharge destination, and f) psychological morbidity. In addition, a manual search of the references of relevant papers was carried out. No limits of year of publication were used but only those in English were included. There was great heterogeneity of the methodology in the studies identified, so a narrative review was performed.

RESULTS

Mortality

Studies which investigate the mortality of delirium in the short and long term have rather inconsistent results. Delirium has been found to be associated with high mortality in elderly patients during hospitalization (Pompei et al. 1994, Francis and Kapoor 1992, Fang et al. 2008) in ICU (e.g. Lin et al. 2004, 2008, Robinson et al. 2009), but not after discharge (Pompei et al. 1994, Levkoff et al. 1992, Francis et al. 1990) while Inouye et al. (1998) reported no association with in-hospital mortality nor at 3 months follow-up. Similarly Villalpando-Berumen et al. (2003) found no difference in mortality during hospitalization, but at 5 year follow-up people who had experienced delirium had higher mortality. Some studies with long follow-up after discharge showed a higher risk for mortality in delirious people (Curyto et al. 2001, Rockwood et al. 1999a, Huang et al. 1998, McCusker et al. 2002, Pitkala et al. 2005, Leslie et al. 2005, Sheng 2006) but others did not (Francis et al. 1990, Francis and Kapoor 1992, O'Keeffe and Lavan 1997, Dolan et al. 2000, Cole et al. 2008a). Similarly inconclusive results have been reported in a more resent systematic review (Siddiqi et al. 2006). The authors reported a wide range of death rates at discharge from 6.1% to 62%.

A meta-analysis (Cole and Primeau 1993) of 8 studies estimated a mortality rate of 14.2% for delirious patients at one month and 22.2% at 6 months and concluded that the presence of dementia or the severity of illness, or both, may have influenced this high rate. In a well-controlled study McCusker et al. (2002) found that 12-month mortality was highest in persons with delirium without pre-existing dementia. This study had a high prevalence of delirium with dementia compared to delirium alone (74% vs. 24%), and in these patients there was a weaker non significant effect of delirium on mortality, even though they had a higher mortality than patients with dementia alone. Perhaps mortality is greater in those with delirium and no pre-existing dementia because in such patients more severe physical illness is required to precipitate a delirium. This contrasts with Francis and Kapoor's finding (1992) in hospitalized delirious patients that mortality risk was largely explained by pre-existing cognitive and functional impairment. In the same line Bellelli et al. (2007) reported that demented patients who had delirium during hospitalization had a increased risk of mortality in the 12 months following discharge than did patients with dementia alone, with delirium alone, or with neither dementia nor delirium. Opposite results reported by Drame et al. (2008) who found that dementia or cognitive impairment did not have any association with death in six weeks time, but delirium had a significant independent association with mortality after controlling for other variables. However there is a possibility that their sample of delirium cases were contaminated with dementia as they assessed dementia from medical files and delirium using the MMSE. When Laurila et al. (2008) re-analyzed their data according to Bellelli et al.'s methodology they found that delirium alone was a significant factor for mortality and not dementia superimposed on delirium (DSD) as Bellelli et al. reported. Cognitive impairment at admission was a strong predictor of later mortality in a study by this author (Adamis et al. (2006)) and in a new prospective study where other biological factors also examined the same group (Adamis et al. 2007) found that delirium was not a predictor of mortality in elderly medical inpatients. Significant predictors associated with death were cognitive impairment, low levels of albumin, higher levels of IFN-γ, and higher levels of IL-6. However in both studies from this group patients with terminal illness were excluded.

Thus the contribution of delirium and dementia (or cognitive impairment) to mortality is complex. Perhaps underling pathophysiological mechanisms common to both delirium and dementia, not detectable by the currently used clinical scales, are related to mortality.

Cognitive Impairment

A number of studies have shown that delirium can cause persistent cognitive impairment. In a prospective study of 70 delirious elderly psychiatric hospitalized patients cognitive deterioration was associated with delirium in 36% of patients at one year follow-up and a non-significant trend was present at 4 years follow-up (Koponen et al. 1989, Koponen and Riekkinen 1993). There appeared to be a survivor effect- patients with more severe cognitive decline died more often during follow up- but most importantly they found that this cognitive decline occurred in patients with CNS disease. Francis and Kapoor (1992) demonstrated in medical inpatients that those who developed delirium had an increased risk of cognitive decline over the next two years. Similarly Rockwood (1993) found prolonged memory impairment in those with delirium, and in a later study (Rockwood et al. 1999a) found that amongst elderly medical inpatients without prior history of dementia an episode of delirium increased the risk of dementia over a median period of 32.5 months follow-up. The unadjusted relative risk of dementia for those with delirium was 3.23 (95% CI 1.86-5.63) and this increased more when it was adjusted for sex, age, and co-morbid illness. Comparable results have been reported by McCusker et al. (2001) who found that delirium is an independent predictor for a later cognitive decline a year after a medical admission to hospital in both patients with, and patients without, pre-existing dementia. Katz et al. (2001) followed up a cohort of 96 people living in care homes (nursing and residential) of whom 47 (49%) were hospitalized at some point during the year of follow-up. Using EEG and a battery of neuropsychological tests they found that subjects who developed delirium were at increased risk of cognitive and decline in cerebral activity (as measured with EEG) during the course of a one-year period. Similar results have been reported by Rahkonen et al. (2000) who followed-up a cohort of healthy community-dwelling subjects without dementia for 2 years;

they found that subjects who developed delirium had a higher than expected incidence of dementia over the two years follow-up period. In an older age group (85 years old and above) they also found similar results (Rahkonen et al. 2001). Two more studies in orthopedic patients (Dolan et al. 2000, Lundström et al. 2003) showed that non-demented patients with preoperative or postoperative delirium had poor cognitive performance or developed dementia during follow-up. Similarly, a systematic review of 13 studies Jackson et al. (2004) concluded that despite methodological problems current research suggests that delirium is associated with an increased risk of subsequent cognitive decline. A very recent review by MacLullich et al. (2009), following the same methodology as Jackson review, evaluated nine reports published after 2004 with a total of 2,025 patients. The authors confirm the previous systematic review that there is a link between delirium and long term cognitive decline.

Fields et al. (1986) examined the effects of delirium on the reversibility of cognition in medically ill inpatients. They found that delirium was not predictive of cognitive improvement but patients with irreversible cognitive deficits were more likely to be rated as demented. No differences were found between those with reversible and non- reversible cognition except that the reversible group had a lower level of cognitive impairment and had lower scores on the Dementia Rating Scale. DSM-III criteria for delirium could not distinguish between the two groups. The authors concluded that the diagnostic criteria commonly associated with reversibility (delirium) are not predictive of the cognitive outcomes, and that there are no ways to predict at admission whose cognitively impaired patients' cognition will improve later.

A recent study (O'Keeffe et al. 2005) suggested that a decline in MMSE score of 2 points is a sensitive (0.93) and specific (0.9) indicator of delirium, and an increase of 3 points or more had a sensitivity of 0.77 and a specificity of 0.75 against improvement of prevalent delirium.

These studies suggest a relationship between delirium and cognitive impairment but there the nature of this association is not clear. If delirium has a poor cognitive outcome itself perhaps the criteria that define delirium are not exclusive of dementia, or pathophysiological mechanisms that are common to both delirium and dementia are responsible for cognitive impairment.

Functional Decline

In a number of studies, delirium in elderly medical inpatients has been associated with increased dependency and functional decline at discharge (e.g. O'Keeffe and Lavan 1997, Inouye et al. 1998, Givens et al. 2008) and at long term follow-up (Francis et al. 1990, Francis and Kapoor 1992, Inouye et al. 1998, McCusker et al. 2001, Bickel et al. 2008). Studies which examined ICU patients e.g. (Balas et al. 2009) have similar findings. In a prospective study of community-dwelling and nursing homes of elderly people who developed incident delirium in hospital delirium was the only independent factor to predict functional decline at 3 months follow-up and this decline was persistent at 6 months after hospital discharge (Murray et al. (1993). Similarly McCusker et al. (2003b) found that those with transient delirium (recovery of delirium within 24h) had better functional outcomes at 12 months follow-up and those with persistent delirium had the worse outcomes, while the recovered group (those who recovered in more than 24h but before discharge) had an intermediate functional outcome. In a study of patients with subsyndromal delirium (SSD) Cole et al. (2003b) also found that patient with SSD had a worse functional outcome at follow-up than patients without any delirious symptoms. In a new study they compared outcomes for 3 groups- those with SSD who recovered, those with SSD who did not recover and those with no SSD symptoms- at 6 and 12 months. They found that the outcomes of the SSD-recovered group were better than the outcomes of the SSD-not recovered group and, intermediate between the outcomes of the SSD-not recovered and no SSD groups Cole et al. (2008b).

In post-acute care settings Marcantonio et al. (2003) reported persistent delirium after the acute hospital discharge which was associated with poor functional recovery. Studies in different medical settings also show a worse functional outcome for patients with delirium. For instance Marcantonio et al. (2000) demonstrated in a study of hip fracture patients that delirium is associated with poor functional outcome, after adjusting for other factors, at 1 month follow-up but not at 6 months. They also reported that those patients whose delirium was still present at 1 month had worse functional outcomes than those whose delirium had resolved. In a later publication from the same cohort Marcantonio et al. (2002) reported that patients with more severe delirium had worse outcomes and the effects of more severe delirium on functional decline were even more evident at 6 months follow-up. Dolan et al.'s study of hip fracture patients also found that those with delirium on admission (preoperative) had worse functional outcomes in subsequent examinations up to 2 years after admission (2000). Edlund et al. (2001) examined patients with hip fracture comparing preoperative with postoperative delirium, and they found that the former had worse outcomes. A retrospective study by Adunsky et al. (2003) also confirmed differences in functional outcome between pre- and postoperative delirious patients.

However not all studies have found an association of delirium with subsequent functional impairment. Pompei et al. (1994) in a mixed population of medical and surgical patients did not find any association of delirium with functional status change between 2 weeks before admission and 3 months after discharge from hospital. Katz et al. (2001) found that hospitalization was associated with functional decline independently of whether the subjects developed delirium during their hospitalization and that it was the medical illness leading to hospitalization that significantly contributed to functional decline. Similar results were reported by Cole et al. (2008a) and Adamis et al. (2006).

The mechanism(s) by which delirium causes long-term disability are not yet known. Given that there is an association between functional decline and cognitive decline it has been suggested (Murray et al. 1993) that delirium may induce a long term or even permanent cognitive decline which then manifests as functional decline. In cases without previous gross cognitive deficits delirium may serve as an early marker of cognitive decline, reflecting low neurological "reserve" (Murray et al. 1993, Francis and Kapoor 1992). Engel and Romano (1959) in their seminal work suggested that delirium may in fact induce brain damage which is irreversible and delirium and dementia could possibly be different stages of the same pathophysiological processes.

Length of Hospital Stay

Prolonged length of stay does not only have implications for the cost of care (Leslie et al. 2008) but also is an increased risk for other hospital-acquired complications. Delirium has been identified as a condition which can prolong hospitalization; and a large number of studies have examined this as a primary or secondary research question. In the literature the results are rather inconsistent. Saravay et al. (1991) and Saravay and Lavin (1994) have identified some methodological flaws in studies which examine length of stay and psychiatric morbidity such as delirium. Studies may be retrospective and based on charts, or based on referrals for liaison psychiatric consultations, often there is not control for severity of medical illness (e.g. Thomas et al. (1988)), they use inappropriate statistical analysis, they lack matched controls or they use psychiatric diagnosis made by physicians.

The most important of studies with the fewer methodological problems will be considered in this review. Inouye et al. (1998) found no difference between delirious and non-delirious inpatients in length of stay after adjusting for age, gender, dementia, illness severity, and functional status. No difference was reported by Ramsay et al. (1991), Jitapunkul et al. (1992), Kolbeinsson and Jonsson (1993), Rockwood (1993), Villalpando-Berumen (2003), while McCusker et al. (2003 a), after controlling for covariates, found that those with incident but not prevalent delirium had prolonged hospital stay. Other studies (e.g. Thomas et al. 1988, Francis et al. 1990, Pompei et al. 1994, Stevens et al. 1998), Thomason et al. (2006), Robinson et al. (2009) (in IC Units) showed a significantly longer hospital stay for delirious people. Those studies which found a longer stay have suggested as reasons: Behavioral problems that accompany delirium, (including falls, the need for restraints and pulling catheters out) (Saravay et al. 2004), severity of physical illness associated with delirium (Thomas et al. 1988), or cognitive impairment (Furlanetto et al. 2003, Fulop et al. 1998). Adamis et al. (2006) found that patients with delirium had a longer hospital stay but this difference was account for mainly by those delirious people who were newly discharged to care homes and who therefore stayed longer than those who were discharged to their previous address. Thus another reason for later hospital discharge of delirious patients may be due to bureaucratic delay (e.g. arrangements for a new place). O'Keeffe and Lavan (1999) reported that delirious patients with hypoactive delirium had longer hospital stays than those with hyperactive or mixed types. Similarly McCusker et al. (2003a) confirmed this after adjusting for covariates, in patients with prevalent or incident delirium. Both groups suggested that patients with hypoactive delirium may stay longer in hospital because they are at higher risk of pressure sores and chest infections, or because it is less likely that hospital staff to detect delirium and treat underlying medical illnesses compared with those with hyperactive delirium. However those with hyperactive delirium are more prone to falls which also has been suggested as a factor for prolonging hospital stay (Saravay et al. 2004).

Discharge Destination

As delirium triggers a cascade of adverse effects (persistent if not permanent) such as cognitive and functional deterioration, perhaps longer hospital stay involves an increased risk of more hospital-acquired disease, A number of studies have also examined new institutionalization after discharge from hospital, and it is not surprising that nearly all have found that delirium is associated with a high rate of institutional care albeit with a few exceptions e.g. Kolbeinsson and Jonsson (1993). Importantly this association has been found in different specialties of medicine, e.g. general medicine (George et al. 1997, Inouye et al. 1998, O'Keeffe and Lavan 1997), orthopedics (Marcantonio et al. 2000, 2002), Givens et al. (2008), Bicker et al. (2008) surgery (Marcantonio et al. 1994), and in ICU (Robinson et al. 2009, Balas et al. 2009) but also in different countries with different health systems like Canada (Cole et al. 1993, Rockwood et al. 1999a), USA (Levkoff et al. 1992, Thomas et al. 1988, McAvay et al. 2006), UK (O'Keeffe and Lavan 1997, Adamis et al. 2006), and Finland (Pitkala et al. 2005). Bourdel-Marchasson et al. (2004) found that SSD -especially incident- was similarly important as full delirium in predicting the institutionalization of elderly medically ill inpatients.

PSYCHOLOGICAL MORBIDITY

It is surprising that only a few studies have examined the psychological impact of delirium in survivors, although some have examined psychological morbidity associated with delirium in the carers and staff. O'Malley et al. (2008) have reviewed studies which examined the psychological morbidity associated with delirium. Symptoms of post traumatic stress disorder have been reported in ICU patients, but in the elderly those symptoms appear to occur less often, (Jones et al. 2007, Roberts et al. 2007, Girard et al. 2007). Feelings of being threatened, anxiety and fear have often been reported in delirious elderly patients. (McCurren and Cronin 2003, Schofield 1997), also feelings of hopelessness, depression and loneliness are common, while very few patients reported that they take pleasure from their delirious experiences. (Schofield 1997, Stenwall et al. 2008). An early study by Breitbart et al. (2002) in cancer patients showed a high level of distress in both spouses/caregivers and nurses caring for delirious patients. Hyperactive delirium and functional disability were strong predictors for spousal distress while perceptual disturbances and severity of delirium were predictors of nursing staff distress. Difficulties in providing adequate care because of delirium also have been reported by Stenwall et al. (2008). Studies which examined the psychological morbidity in elderly patients but also the psychological impact on caregivers and nurses are few. This area needs further investigation to provide new hypotheses and suggestions for therapeutic approaches and better management of delirium for each individual patient (O'Malley et al. 2008).

Discussion

As in previous reviews (Jackson 2004, Siddiqi et al. 2006, MacLullich et al. 2009), there are inconsistent findings in some of the delirium outcomes and the studies examined have different methodologies, designs and patient populations and often inadequate sample sizes.

Mortality

The results of studies of the relationship of delirium to mortality during hospitalization, but also at long term follow up, are contradictory. A possible explanation for this is that nearly all studies suffer lack of power to detect true differences. Furthermore studies which investigated the long term mortality inevitably included patients newly discarded to care homes. If delirium is a factor for institutionalization, more people with delirium will be discharged to care homes compared to non delirious people. Studies also show that in those newly admitted to care homes there are high mortality rates (e.g. Aneshensel et al. 2000, van Dijk et al. 1992, Shapiro and Tate 1988). Suggested reasons for this have included those of social causation (that the institutionalization is the direct cause of death) and of social selection (that the decline in health and proximity to death produce relocation and death) (Aneshensel et al. 2000). Thus perhaps institutionalization is a more important factor related to mortality -in long term follow up- than delirium itself.

There is a possibility that biological factors like IL-6, C-RP, albumin may play a role in mortality and although some of these are already known, (e.g. Roubenoff et al. 2003, Evrin et al. 2005) they need to be taken into account when trying to understand the sequelae of an episode of delirium during acute illness in hospital. A number of studies have shown that previous cognitive impairment and dementia are predictors of later mortality. Thus perhaps delirium and dementia share common pathophysiological pathways which are related to mortality and which the currently-used methods cannot detect.

Cognitive Impairment

Nearly all studies but and previous systematic reviews show a relationship between delirium and subsequent cognitive decline in elderly inpatients. (Jackson 2004, Siddiqi et al. 2006, MacLullich et al. 2009). A number of explanations have been proposed for this relation (MacLullich et al. 2009). Delirium may not be causally related to cognitive decline but a marker of its progression; an epiphenomenon. Perhaps delirium is a consequence of acute brain damage which is also responsible for triggering a cascade of active processes causing cognitive decline. It is also possible that delirium is a cause of cognitive decline; alternatively medications used to treat delirium may be causal of cognitive decline. All of those suggested reasons remain speculative. There may be a combination of the above mechanism with genetic factors. Indeed a study (Adamis 2007 thesis) found that variables that significantly influence cognitive impairment are IGF-I, the severity of delirium, the age of the subject, and the interaction of the APOE genotype with the severity of delirium, but only in those who do not carry the APOE epsilon 4 allele.

Functional Decline

Not all studies have found an association of delirium and consequent functional decline. A number of reasons can be suggested for discrepancies in the literature. Firstly, several studies use premorbid measurements of functional ability relying on informants or patients (e.g. Murray et al. 1993, Inouye et al. 1998, Marcantonio et al. 2000), although it is known that patients overestimate their functional ability while proxies underestimate it (Magaziner et al. 1997, Magaziner 1997). Secondly, premorbid measurement does not usually include states immediately after the illness that precipitated the admission, which can contribute significantly to deterioration in function. Thirdly, some studies are disadvantaged where they present differences between subjects but not within subjects (e.g. McCusker et al. 2001). Large studies like that of Inouye et al. (1998) used data from different hospitals to increase the power of the study, but although they controlled for other variables they did not control for hospitals. It is widely accepted that institutional and environmental factors can contribute significantly not only to the genesis of delirium but also its recognition, treatment and rehabilitation. For instance, a study by Esperanza et al. (2004) demonstrated that better outcomes for patients with delirium can be achieved in specific rehabilitation units. Finally, a number of studies have long follow up periods and measure long-term functional outcomes (2 years), (e.g. Francis and Kapoor 1992, Dolan et al. 2000) and although they control for initial confounding variables, they cannot control for any new variables during the follow up period which may have an influence on the functional ability, e.g. new onset of illness.

Some other underlying biological factors may play a role in functional decline, together or independently of delirium status, which may explain these discrepancies. Indeed a number of studies which examined APOE genotype have found an association between possession of the epsilon 4 allele and worse functional outcome in patients with brain injuries and intracerebral hemorrhage (e.g. Alberts et al. 1995, Greenberg et al. 1996, McCarron et al. 1998, 2003 Teasdale et al. 1997). Similarly a study by El Solh et al. 2006 showed that higher serum levels of TNF-α were a risk for functional impairment for hospitalized elderly patients with community –acquired pneumonia. In our study (Adamis 2007 thesis) the important factors associated with functional decline were cognitive impairment, APOE genotype, and the levels of the cytokines IL-1α, IL-6, TNF-α, and LIF. However those findings need to be confirmed in other studies. It seems important that future studies need to investigate both biological factors that may be responsible for functional decline as well as phenomenology.

Length of Hospital Stay

As reported above there is no general agreement on whether delirium is an independent factor prolonging stay in hospital. As well as different methodologies and settings other confounding factors needs to be controlled for. Perhaps other reasons like completing paper-work, approval for placement etc. influenced length of stay in hospital much more than delirium per se. Other related factors may include socio-economic status, different hospital policies, demands for bed and time of the year.

Discharge Destination

In contrast, nearly all studies found that delirium is a condition which is responsible for relocation in care homes. This may be due to cognitive or functional decline or both but there is a possibility that it is due to persistent delirium. It is also highly likely that factors other than delirium play a role in placement including seasonal differences and consequent changes in pressure on hospitals beds, availability of care home beds or changes in local policies and funding arrangements. Not all of those factors, many of which apply to comparisons between studies from different centers and times, have been examined in the studies reviewed and no definitive assertion is possible.

Psychological Morbidity

Although there is unanimity that delirium is a very distressing syndrome to patients, carers and nursing staff, with sort and long term psychological stress and impact on wellbeing, very few studies, especially those of the elderly, have examined this outcome. For example, there is no evidence yet of the benefits or risks of discussion about the experiences that people had during delirium. Further studies of this underesearched area are needed.

Subsyndromal Delirium

As the new notion of SSD is emerging a number of studies which investigate its outcomes have been published. Marcantonio et al. (2002) investigated the outcomes for elderly patients after surgery of acute hip fracture and they found that subjects who did not meet the full criteria of delirium (as assessed with CAM) experienced worse outcomes than those who had no or fewer symptoms. Cole et al. (2003b) confirmed previous studies and concluded that SSD in elderly medical patients is an important concept. Subsyndromal presentations have been also suggested for other clinical diagnoses and Royall (2004), who is in favor of subsyndromal presentations as validated by clinical outcomes intermediate between no pathology and the full clinical syndrome, cautioned that the linear association between the severity of the symptoms in question and clinical outcomes needs to be established. It seems that more research is necessary to establish the exact significance of SSD but it is sufficient to note that categorical diagnoses have their limitations. Nevertheless DSM-IV does recognize subclinical presentations of delirium without explicitly indicating if they are prodromal, never progress to delirium (SSD) or part of the recovery from delirium; it suggests that all of them can be coded as cognitive disorders not otherwise specified.

Definition of Delirium According to its Course and Outcome

Diagnostic criteria for delirium in both international classification systems are mainly focused on presenting symptoms, with little emphasis on the course of the disorder, although the ICD-10 does take in to account duration of symptoms in distinguishing delirium from dementia. Historically major steps in psychiatric understanding have followed longitudinal observations. Kraepelin (1899) for instance distinguished manic-depression from schizophrenia mainly on the basis of differences in the course of illness and the outcome. The relative absence of outcome criteria in the definition of delirium is understandable because if it cannot be defined until the outcome is known (perhaps when the illness itself has disappeared) the definition has little or no clinical significance (Macdonald and Treloar 1996). Conversely, ignoring outcome makes it difficult to distinguish delirium from other cognitive disorders especially dementia with which they share many common characteristics (Lindesay et al. 1990). One group has proposed that reversibility of cognition should be a criterion for the definition of delirium (Treloar and Macdonald 1997a, b). Another solution may be to distinguish different subtypes of delirium based on clinical and biochemical criteria which are present at first assessment and which can predict outcome (Macdonald 1999).

CONCLUSIONS

From the above it is clear that delirium has very serious adverse outcomes and it is necessary to develop scales and biological markers which can allow a focus of preventative measures on those at most risk of developing this distressing, dangerous and only sometimes reversible syndrome. In addition by using biological methods to identify those at risk we may be able to alter or block those biological pathways with pharmacological or other interventions to protect patients from these unfavorable outcomes.

REFERENCES

Adamis, D. (2007). *APOE and cytokines as biological markers of recovery of delirium in elderly medical inpatients.* University of London, London.

Adamis, D., Treloar, A., Darwiche, F. Z., Gregson, N., Macdonald, A. J., and Martin, F. C. (2007). Associations of delirium with in-hospital and in 6-months mortality in elderly medical inpatients. *Age Ageing, 36*(6), 644-649.

Adamis, D., Treloar, A., Martin, F. C., and Macdonald, A. J. (2006). Recovery and outcome of delirium in elderly medical inpatients. *Arch Gerontol Geriatr, 43*(2), 289-298.

Adunsky, A., Levy, R., Heim, M., Mizrahi, E., and Arad, M. (2003). The unfavorable nature of preoperative delirium in elderly hip fractured patients. *Arch Gerontol Geriatr, 36*(1), 67-74.

Alberts, M. J., Graffagnino, C., McClenny, C., DeLong, D., Strittmatter, W., Saunders, A. M., et al. (1995). ApoE genotype and survival from intracerebral haemorrhage. *Lancet, 346*(8974), 575.

American Psychiatric Association Task Force on, D.-I. (1994). *DSM-IV : diagnostic and statistical manual of mental disorders* (4th ed ed.). Washington, D.C.: American Psychiatric Association.

Aneshensel, C. S., Pearlin, L. I., Levy-Storms, L., and Schuler, R. H. (2000). The transition from home to nursing home mortality among people with dementia. *J Gerontol B Psychol Sci Soc Sci, 55*(3), S152-162.

Balas, M. C., Happ, M. B., Yang, W., Chelluri, L., and Richmond, T. (2009). Outcomes Associated With Delirium in Older Patients in Surgical ICUs. *Chest, 135*(1), 18-25.

Bedford, P. D. (1959). General medical aspects of confusional states in elderly people. *Br Med J, 2*(5145), 185-188.

Bellelli, G., Speciale, S., Barisione, E., and Trabucchi, M. (2007). Delirium subtypes and 1-year mortality among elderly patients discharged from a post-acute rehabilitation facility. *J Gerontol A Biol Sci Med Sci, 62*(10), 1182-1183.

Bickel, H., Gradinger, R., Kochs, E., and Forstl, H. (2008). High risk of cognitive and functional decline after postoperative delirium. A three-year prospective study. *Dement Geriatr Cogn Disord, 26*(1), 26-31.

Bleuler, M., Willi, J., and Bühler, H. R. (1966). *Akute psychische Begleiterscheinungen köperlicher Krankheiten.* Stuttgart,: G. Thieme.

Bourdel-Marchasson, I., Vincent, S., Germain, C., Salles, N., Jenn, J., Rasoamanarivo, E., et al. (2004). Delirium symptoms and low dietary intake in older inpatients are independent predictors of institutionalization: a 1-year prospective population-based study. *J Gerontol A Biol Sci Med Sci, 59*(4), 350-354.

Breitbart, W., Gibson, C., and Tremblay, A. (2002). The delirium experience: delirium recall and delirium-related distress in hospitalized patients with cancer, their spouses/caregivers, and their nurses. *Psychosomatics, 43*(3), 183-194.

Chisholm, S. E., Deniston, O. L., Igrisan, R. M., and Barbus, A. J. (1982). Prevalence of confusion in elderly hospitalized patients. *J Gerontol Nurs, 8*(2), 87-96.

Cole, M., McCusker, J., Dendukuri, N., and Han, L. (2003b). The prognostic significance of subsyndromal delirium in elderly medical inpatients. *J Am Geriatr Soc, 51*(6), 754-760.

Cole, M. G., Dendukuri, N., McCusker, J., and Han, L. (2003a). An empirical study of different diagnostic criteria for delirium among elderly medical inpatients. *J Neuropsychiatry Clin Neurosci, 15*(2), 200-207.

Cole, M. G., McCusker, J., Bellavance, F., Primeau, F. J., Bailey, R. F., Bonnycastle, M. J., et al. (2002). Systematic detection and multidisciplinary care of delirium in older medical inpatients: a randomized trial. *Cmaj, 167*(7), 753-759.

Cole, M. G., McCusker, J., Ciampi, A., and Belzile, E. (2008b). The 6- and 12-month outcomes of older medical inpatients who recover from subsyndromal delirium. *J Am Geriatr Soc, 56*(11), 2093-2099.

Cole, M. G., and Primeau, F. J. (1993). Prognosis of delirium in elderly hospital patients. *Cmaj, 149*(1), 41-46.

Cole, M. G., You, Y., McCusker, J., Ciampi, A., and Belzile, E. (2008a). The 6 and 12 month outcomes of older medical inpatients who recover from delirium. *Int J Geriatr Psychiatry, 23*(3), 301-307.

Cooper, J. E., and World Health, O. (1994). *Pocket guide to the ICD-10 classification of mental and behavioural disorders*. Edinburgh: Churchill Livingstone.

Curyto, K. J., Johnson, J., TenHave, T., Mossey, J., Knott, K., and Katz, I. R. (2001). Survival of hospitalized elderly patients with delirium: a prospective study. *Am J Geriatr Psychiatry, 9*(2), 141-147.

Dolan, M. M., Hawkes, W. G., Zimmerman, S. I., Morrison, R. S., Gruber-Baldini, A. L., Hebel, J. R., et al. (2000). Delirium on hospital admission in aged hip fracture patients: Prediction of mortality and 2-year functional outcomes. *Journals of Gerontology Series a-Biological Sciences and Medical Sciences, 55*(9), M527-M534.

Drame, M., Jovenin, N., Novella, J. L., Lang, P. O., Somme, D., Laniece, I., et al. (2008). Predicting early mortality among elderly patients hospitalised in medical wards via emergency department: the SAFES cohort study. *J Nutr Health Aging, 12*(8), 599-604.

Edlund, A., Lundstrom, M., Brannstrom, B., Bucht, G., and Gustafson, Y. (2001). Delirium before and after operation for femoral neck fracture. *J Am Geriatr Soc, 49*(10), 1335-1340.

El Solh, A., Pineda, L., Bouquin, P., and Mankowski, C. (2006). Determinants of short and long term functional recovery after hospitalization for community-acquired pneumonia in the elderly: role of inflammatory markers. *BMC Geriatr, 6*, 12.

Engel, G. L., and Romano, J. (1959). Delirium, a syndrome of cerebral insufficiency. *J Chronic Dis, 9*(3), 260-277.

Esperanza, A., Miralles, R., Rius, I., Fernandez, B., Digon, A., Arranz, P., et al. (2004). Evaluation of functional improvement in older patients with cognitive impairment, depression and/or delirium admitted to a geriatric convalescence hospitalization unit. *Arch Gerontol Geriatr Suppl*(9), 149-153.

Evrin, P. E., Nilsson, S. E., Oberg, T., and Malmberg, B. (2005). Serum C-reactive protein in elderly men and women: association with mortality, morbidity and various biochemical values. *Scand J Clin Lab Invest, 65*(1), 23-31.

Fang, C. K., Chen, H. W., Liu, S. I., Lin, C. J., Tsai, L. Y., and Lai, Y. L. (2008). Prevalence, detection and treatment of delirium in terminal cancer inpatients: a prospective survey. *Jpn J Clin Oncol, 38*(1), 56-63.

Fields, S. D., MacKenzie, C. R., Charlson, M. E., and Perry, S. W. (1986). Reversibility of cognitive impairment in medical inpatients. *Arch Intern Med, 146*(8), 1593-1596.

Flint, F. J., and Richards, S. M. (1956). Organic basis of confusional states in the elderly. *Br Med J, 2*(5008), 1537-1539.

Francis, J., and Kapoor, W. N. (1992). Prognosis after hospital discharge of older medical patients with delirium. *J Am Geriatr Soc, 40*(6), 601-606.

Francis, J., Martin, D., and Kapoor, W. N. (1990). A prospective study of delirium in hospitalized elderly. *Jama, 263*(8), 1097-1101.

Fulop, G., Strain, J. J., Fahs, M. C., Schmeidler, J., and Snyder, S. (1998). A prospective study of the impact of psychiatric comorbidity on length of hospital stays of elderly medical-surgical inpatients. *Psychosomatics, 39*(3), 273-280.

Furlanetto, L. M., da Silva, R. V., and Bueno, J. R. (2003). The impact of psychiatric comorbidity on length of stay of medical inpatients. *Gen Hosp Psychiatry, 25*(1), 14-19.

George, J., Bleasdale, S., and Singleton, S. J. (1997). Causes and prognosis of delirium in elderly patients admitted to a district general hospital. *Age Ageing, 26*(6), 423-427.

Girard, T. D., Shintani, A. K., Jackson, J. C., Gordon, S. M., Pun, B. T., Henderson, M. S., et al. (2007). Risk factors for post-traumatic stress disorder symptoms following critical illness requiring mechanical ventilation: a prospective cohort study. *Crit Care, 11*(1), R28.

Givens, J. L., Sanft, T. B., and Marcantonio, E. R. (2008). Functional recovery after hip fracture: the combined effects of depressive symptoms, cognitive impairment, and delirium. *J Am Geriatr Soc, 56*(6), 1075-1079.

Greenberg, S. M., Briggs, M. E., Hyman, B. T., Kokoris, G. J., Takis, C., Kanter, D. S., et al. (1996). Apolipoprotein E epsilon 4 is associated with the presence and earlier onset of hemorrhage in cerebral amyloid angiopathy. *Stroke, 27*(8), 1333-1337.

Hodkinson, H. M. (1973). Mental impairment in the elderly. *J R Coll Physicians Lond, 7*(4), 305-317.

Inouye, S. K., Rushing, J. T., Foreman, M. D., Palmer, R. M., and Pompei, P. (1998). Does delirium contribute to poor hospital outcomes? A three-site epidemiologic study. *J Gen Intern Med, 13*(4), 234-242.

Inouye, S. K., Viscoli, C. M., Horwitz, R. I., Hurst, L. D., and Tinetti, M. E. (1993). A predictive model for delirium in hospitalized elderly medical patients based on admission characteristics. *Ann Intern Med, 119*(6), 474-481.

Jackson, J. C., Gordon, S. M., Hart, R. P., Hopkins, R. O., and Ely, E. W. (2004). The association between delirium and cognitive decline: a review of the empirical literature. *Neuropsychol Rev, 14*(2), 87-98.

Jitapunkul, S., Pillay, I., and Ebrahim, S. (1992). Delirium in newly admitted elderly patients: a prospective study. *Q J Med, 83*(300), 307-314.

Jones, C., Backman, C., Capuzzo, M., Flaatten, H., Rylander, C., and Griffiths, R. D. (2007). Precipitants of post-traumatic stress disorder following intensive care: a hypothesis generating study of diversity in care. *Intensive Care Med, 33*(6), 978-985.

Katz, I. R., Curyto, K. J., TenHave, T., Mossey, J., Sands, L., and Kallan, M. J. (2001). Validating the diagnosis of delirium and evaluating its association with deterioration over a one-year period. *Am J Geriatr Psychiatry, 9*(2), 148-159.

Kolbeinsson, H., and Jonsson, A. (1993). Delirium and dementia in acute medical admissions of elderly patients in Iceland. *Acta Psychiatr Scand, 87*(2), 123-127.

Koponen, H., Stenback, U., Mattila, E., Soininen, H., Reinikainen, K., and Riekkinen, P. J. (1989). Delirium among elderly persons admitted to a psychiatric hospital: clinical course during the acute stage and one-year follow-up. *Acta Psychiatr Scand, 79*(6), 579-585.

Koponen, H. J., and Riekkinen, P. J. (1993). A prospective study of delirium in elderly patients admitted to a psychiatric hospital. *Psychol Med, 23*(1), 103-109.

Korevaar, J. C., van Munster, B. C., and de Rooij, S. E. (2005). Risk factors for delirium in acutely admitted elderly patients: a prospective cohort study. *BMC Geriatr, 5*, 6.

Kraepelin, E. (1899). *Psychiatrie : ein Lehrbuch für Studirende und Aerzte* (6. vollständig umgearb. Aufl ed.). Leipzig: J.A. Barth.

Laurila, J. V., Pitkala, K. H., Strandberg, T. E., and Tilvis, R. S. (2004). Detection and documentation of dementia and delirium in acute geriatric wards. *Gen Hosp Psychiatry, 26*(1), 31-35.

Laurila, J. V., Pitkala, K. H., Strandberg, T. E., and Tilvis, R. S. (2008). Delirium superimposed on dementia predicts 12-month survival in elderly patients discharged from a postacute rehabilitation facility: a comment. *J Gerontol A Biol Sci Med Sci, 63*(10), 1124-1125; author reply 1125-1126.

Leentjens, A. F., Maclullich, A. M., and Meagher, D. J. (2008). Delirium, Cinderella no more...? *J Psychosom Res, 65*(3), 205.

Leslie, D. L., Marcantonio, E. R., Zhang, Y., Leo-Summers, L., and Inouye, S. K. (2008). One-year health care costs associated with delirium in the elderly population. *Arch Intern Med, 168*(1), 27-32.

Leslie, D. L., Zhang, Y., Holford, T. R., Bogardus, S. T., Leo-Summers, L. S., and Inouye, S. K. (2005). Premature death associated with delirium at 1-year follow-up. *Arch Intern Med, 165*(14), 1657-1662.

Levkoff, S., Frances, S., Yang, M., and Liptzin, B. (2004). Delirium: The Importance of Subsyndromal States. *Primary Psychiatry., 11*(11), 40-44.

Levkoff, S., Liptzin, B., Cleary, P., Wetle, T., Evans, D., Rowe, J., et al. (1996). Subsyndromal delirium. *American Journal of Geriatric Psychiatry, 4*(4), 320-329.

Levkoff, S. E., Evans, D. A., Liptzin, B., Cleary, P. D., Lipsitz, L. A., Wetle, T. T., et al. (1992). Delirium. The occurrence and persistence of symptoms among elderly hospitalized patients. *Arch Intern Med, 152*(2), 334-340.

Lin, S. M., Huang, C. D., Liu, C. Y., Lin, H. C., Wang, C. H., Huang, P. Y., et al. (2008). Risk factors for the development of early-onset delirium and the subsequent clinical outcome in mechanically ventilated patients. *J Crit Care, 23*(3), 372-379.

Lin, S. M., Liu, C. Y., Wang, C. H., Lin, H. C., Huang, C. D., Huang, P. Y., et al. (2004). The impact of delirium on the survival of mechanically ventilated patients. *Crit Care Med, 32*(11), 2254-2259.

Lindesay, J., Macdonald, A., and Starke, I. (1990). *Delirium in the elderly*. Oxford ; New York: Oxford University Press.

Lindesay, J., Rockwood, K., and Macdonald, A. (2002). *Delirium in old age*. Oxford ; New York: Oxford University Press.

Lundstrom, M., Edlund, A., Bucht, G., Karlsson, S., and Gustafson, Y. (2003). Dementia after delirium in patients with femoral neck fractures. *J Am Geriatr Soc, 51*(7), 1002-1006.

Macdonald, A. J. (1999). Can delirium be separated from dementia? *Dement Geriatr Cogn Disord, 10*(5), 386-388.

Macdonald, A. J., and Treloar, A. (1996). Delirium and dementia; are they distinct? *J Am Geriatr Soc, 44*(8), 1001-1002.

MacLullich, A. M., Beaglehole, A., Hall, R. J., and Meagher, D. J. (2009). Delirium and long-term cognitive impairment. *Int Rev Psychiatry, 21*(1), 30-42.

Magaziner, J. (1997). Use of proxies to measure health and functional outcomes in effectiveness research in persons with Alzheimer disease and related disorders. *Alzheimer Dis Assoc Disord, 11 Suppl 6*, 168-174.

Magaziner, J., Zimmerman, S. I., Gruber-Baldini, A. L., Hebel, J. R., and Fox, K. M. (1997). Proxy reporting in five areas of functional status. Comparison with self-reports and observations of performance. *Am J Epidemiol, 146*(5), 418-428.

Marcantonio, E., Ta, T., Duthie, E., and Resnick, N. M. (2002). Delirium severity and psychomotor types: their relationship with outcomes after hip fracture repair. *J Am Geriatr Soc, 50*(5), 850-857.

Marcantonio, E. R., Flacker, J. M., Michaels, M., and Resnick, N. M. (2000). Delirium is independently associated with poor functional recovery after hip fracture. *Journal of the American Geriatrics Society, 48*(6), 618-624.

Marcantonio, E. R., Goldman, L., Mangione, C. M., Ludwig, L. E., Muraca, B., Haslauer, C. M., et al. (1994). A clinical prediction rule for delirium after elective noncardiac surgery. *Jama, 271*(2), 134-139.

Marcantonio, E. R., Simon, S. E., Bergmann, M. A., Jones, R. N., Murphy, K. M., and Morris, J. N. (2003). Delirium symptoms in post-acute care: Prevalent, persistent, and associated with poor functional recovery. *Journal of the American Geriatrics Society, 51*(1), 4-9.

McAvay, G. J., Van Ness, P. H., Bogardus, S. T., Jr., Zhang, Y., Leslie, D. L., Leo-Summers, L. S., et al. (2006). Older adults discharged from the hospital with delirium: 1-year outcomes. *J Am Geriatr Soc, 54*(8), 1245-1250.

McCarron, M., Muir, K. W., Weir, C. J., Dyker, A. G., Bone, I., Nicoll, J. A., et al. (1998). The apolipoprotein E epsilon4 allele and outcome in cerebrovascular disease. *Stroke, 29*(9), 1882-1887.

McCarron, M. O., Weir, C. J., Muir, K. W., Hoffmann, K. L., Graffagnino, C., Nicoll, J. A., et al. (2003). Effect of apolipoprotein E genotype on in-hospital mortality following intracerebral haemorrhage. *Acta Neurol Scand, 107*(2), 106-109.

McCurren, C., and Cronin, S. N. (2003). Delirium: elders tell their stories and guide nursing practice. *Medsurg Nurs, 12*(5), 318-323.

McCusker, J., Cole, M., Abrahamowicz, M., Primeau, F., and Belzile, E. (2002). Delirium predicts 12-month mortality. *Arch Intern Med, 162*(4), 457-463.

McCusker, J., Cole, M., Dendukuri, N., Belzile, E., and Primeau, F. (2001). Delirium in older medical inpatients and subsequent cognitive and functional status: a prospective study. *Cmaj, 165*(5), 575-583.

McCusker, J., Cole, M., Dendukuri, N., Han, L., and Belzile, E. (2003b). The course of delirium in older medical inpatients: a prospective study. *J Gen Intern Med, 18*(9), 696-704.

McCusker, J., Cole, M. G., Dendukuri, N., and Belzile, E. (2003a). Does delirium increase hospital stay? *J Am Geriatr Soc, 51*(11), 1539-1546.

Murray, A. M., Levkoff, S. E., Wetle, T. T., Beckett, L., Cleary, P. D., Schor, J. D., et al. (1993). Acute delirium and functional decline in the hospitalized elderly patient. *J Gerontol, 48*(5), M181-186.

Naughton, B. J., Saltzman, S., Ramadan, F., Chadha, N., Priore, R., and Mylotte, J. M. (2005). A multifactorial intervention to reduce prevalence of delirium and shorten hospital length of stay. *J Am Geriatr Soc, 53*(1), 18-23.

O'Keeffe, S., and Lavan, J. (1997). The prognostic significance of delirium in older hospital patients. *J Am Geriatr Soc, 45*(2), 174-178.

O'Keeffe, S. T., and Lavan, J. N. (1999). Clinical significance of delirium subtypes in older people. *Age Ageing, 28*(2), 115-119.

O'Keeffe, S. T., Mulkerrin, E. C., Nayeem, K., Varughese, M., and Pillay, I. (2005). Use of serial Mini-Mental State Examinations to diagnose and monitor delirium in elderly hospital patients. *J Am Geriatr Soc, 53*(5), 867-870.

O'Malley, G., Leonard, M., Meagher, D., and O'Keeffe, S. T. (2008). The delirium experience: a review. *J Psychosom Res, 65*(3), 223-228.

Pandharipande, P., Cotton, B. A., Shintani, A., Thompson, J., Pun, B. T., Morris, J. A., Jr., et al. (2008). Prevalence and risk factors for development of delirium in surgical and trauma intensive care unit patients. *J Trauma, 65*(1), 34-41.

Pitkala, K. H., Laurila, J. V., Strandberg, T. E., and Tilvis, R. S. (2005). Prognostic significance of delirium in frail older people. *Dement Geriatr Cogn Disord, 19*(2-3), 158-163.

Pompei, P., Foreman, M., Rudberg, M. A., Inouye, S. K., Braund, V., and Cassel, C. K. (1994). Delirium in hospitalized older persons: outcomes and predictors. *J Am Geriatr Soc, 42*(8), 809-815.

Rahkonen, T., Eloniemi-Sulkava, U., Halonen, P., Verkkoniemi, A., Niinisto, L., Notkola, I. L., et al. (2001). Delirium in the non-demented oldest old in the general population: risk factors and prognosis. *Int J Geriatr Psychiatry, 16*(4), 415-421.

Rahkonen, T., Luukkainen-Markkula, R., Paanila, S., Sivenius, J., and Sulkava, R. (2000). Delirium episode as a sign of undetected dementia among community dwelling elderly subjects: a 2 year follow up study. *J Neurol Neurosurg Psychiatry, 69*(4), 519-521.

Ramsay, R., Wright, P., Katz, A., Bielawska, C., and Katona, C. (1991). The detection of psychiatric morbidity and its effects on outcome in acute elderly medical admissions. *International Journal of Geriatric Psychiatry, 6*, 861-866.

Roberts, B. L., Rickard, C. M., Rajbhandari, D., and Reynolds, P. (2007). Factual memories of ICU: recall at two years post-discharge and comparison with delirium status during ICU admission--a multicentre cohort study. *J Clin Nurs, 16*(9), 1669-1677.

Robinson, T. N., Raeburn, C. D., Tran, Z. V., Angles, E. M., Brenner, L. A., and Moss, M. (2009). Postoperative delirium in the elderly: risk factors and outcomes. *Ann Surg, 249*(1), 173-178.

Rockwood, K. (1993). The occurrence and duration of symptoms in elderly patients with delirium. *J Gerontol, 48*(4), M162-166.

Rockwood, K., Cosway, S., Carver, D., Jarrett, P., Stadnyk, K., and Fisk, J. (1999). The risk of dementia and death after delirium. *Age Ageing, 28*(6), 551-556.

Roubenoff, R., Parise, H., Payette, H. A., Abad, L. W., D'Agostino, R., Jacques, P. F., et al. (2003). Cytokines, insulin-like growth factor 1, sarcopenia, and mortality in very old community-dwelling men and women: the Framingham Heart Study. *Am J Med, 115*(6), 429-435.

Royall, D. R. (2004). The "subsyndromal" syndromes of aging. *J Am Geriatr Soc, 52*(3), 463-465.

Saravay, S. M., Kaplowitz, M., Kurek, J., Zeman, D., Pollack, S., Novik, S., et al. (2004). How do delirium and dementia increase length of stay of elderly general medical inpatients? *Psychosomatics, 45*(3), 235-242.

Saravay, S. M., and Lavin, M. (1994). Psychiatric comorbidity and length of stay in the general hospital. A critical review of outcome studies. *Psychosomatics, 35*(3), 233-252.

Saravay, S. M., Steinberg, M. D., Weinschel, B., Pollack, S., and Alovis, N. (1991). Psychological comorbidity and length of stay in the general hospital. *Am J Psychiatry, 148*(3), 324-329.

Schmidt, N. B., Kotov, R., and Joiner, T. E. (2004). *Taxometrics : toward a new diagnostic scheme for psychopathology*. Washington, DC ; London: American Psychological Association.

Schofield, I. (1997). A small exploratory study of the reaction of older people to an episode of delirium. *J Adv Nurs, 25*(5), 942-952.

Shapiro, E., and Tate, R. (1988). Survival patterns of nursing home admissions and their policy implications. *Can J Public Health, 79*(4), 268-274.

Sheng, A. Z., Shen, Q., Cordato, D., Zhang, Y. Y., and Yin Chan, D. K. (2006). Delirium within three days of stroke in a cohort of elderly patients. *J Am Geriatr Soc, 54*(8), 1192-1198.

Siddiqi, N., House, A. O., and Holmes, J. D. (2006). Occurrence and outcome of delirium in medical in-patients: a systematic literature review. *Age Ageing, 35*(4), 350-364.

Simon, A., and Cahan, R. (1963). The acute brain syndrome in geriatric patients. *Psychiatric Research Reports, 16*, 8-21.

Stenwall, E., Jonhagen, M. E., Sandberg, J., and Fagerberg, I. (2008). The older patient's experience of encountering professional carers and close relatives during an acute confusional state: an interview study. *Int J Nurs Stud, 45*(11), 1577-1585.

Stevens, L. E., de Moore, G. M., and Simpson, J. M. (1998). Delirium in hospital: does it increase length of stay? *Aust N Z J Psychiatry, 32*(6), 805-808.

Teasdale, G. M., Nicoll, J. A., Murray, G., and Fiddes, M. (1997). Association of apolipoprotein E polymorphism with outcome after head injury. *Lancet, 350*(9084), 1069-1071.

Thomas, R. I., Cameron, D. J., and Fahs, M. C. (1988). A prospective study of delirium and prolonged hospital stay. Exploratory study. *Arch Gen Psychiatry, 45*(10), 937-940.

Thomason, J. W., Shintani, A., Peterson, J. F., Pun, B. T., Jackson, J. C., and Ely, E. W. (2005). Intensive care unit delirium is an independent predictor of longer hospital stay: a prospective analysis of 261 non-ventilated patients. *Crit Care, 9*(4), R375-381.

Treloar, A. J., and Macdonald, A. J. (1997a). Outcome of delirium: Part 1. Outcome of delirium diagnosed by DSM-III-R, ICD-10 and CAMDEX and derivation of the

Reversible Cognitive Dysfunction Scale among acute geriatric inpatients. *Int J Geriatr Psychiatry, 12*(6), 609-613.

Treloar, A. J., and Macdonald, A. J. (1997b). Outcome of delirium: part 2. Clinical features of reversible cognitive dysfunction--are they the same as accepted definitions of delirium? *Int J Geriatr Psychiatry, 12*(6), 614-618.

van Dijk, P. T., van de Sande, H. J., Dippel, D. W., and Habbema, J. D. (1992). The nature of excess mortality in nursing home patients with dementia. *J Gerontol, 47*(2), M28-34.

Villalpando-Berumen, J. M., Pineda-Colorado, A. M., Palacios, P., Reyes-Guerrero, J., Villa, A. R., and Gutierrez-Robledo, L. M. (2003). Incidence of delirium, risk factors, and long-term survival of elderly patients hospitalized in a medical specialty teaching hospital in Mexico City. *Int Psychogeriatr, 15*(4), 325-336.

In: Psychiatric Research Trends: Dreams and Geriatric Psychiatry ISBN 978-1-60741-760-6
Editors: Daniella M. Montez, pp.67-78

Chapter 4

LATE-LIFE ANXIETY IN THE ELDERLY

Gary Sinoff
Department of Geriatrics, Carmel Medical Center, Technion Medical School,
The Technion Institute of Technology, Haifa, Israel

ABSTRACT

Anxiety as a separate disorder was introduced into the DSM manuals only in 1980, but is now widely recognized as a common mood disorder in the elderly, and in fact its prevalence, reported to range between 10% to 20% may actually be greater than for depressive illness. On the other hand, its assessment and diagnosis is problematic, and therefore, frequently often under-recognized. Conversely, though the elderly may not actually meet the full requirements for anxiety disorder, they still experience enough symptoms which can disrupt their daily lives. The problem is complicated by the fact that elderly persons have a high incidence of somatic symptoms accompanying their physical illnesses, and also that anxiety in the elderly presents with somatic complaints, then their complaints may be interpreted as being part of some physical illness rather than actually been related to their anxiety, somewhat similar to the problem in diagnosing depression in the elderly. Similarly to depression, several screening instruments were developed and validated for the detection of anxiety, but rarely specifically for the elderly. This chapter will describe and define late-life anxiety, the means of diagnosing the disorder relating especially to the difficulties in the elderly, and finally its interaction with depression.

INTRODUCTION

Though anxiety as a separate disorder was only introduced into the third edition of the *Diagnostic and Statistical Manual of Mental Disorders* published in 1980, it is now widely recognized as a common mood disorder and is especially prevalent in the elderly [Joormann, & Stöber, 1999; Lenze, & Wetherell, 2008]. In a Medline search using the key words late-life and anxiety, two hundred and ten articles were listed of which 207 were since 1990, emphasizing its increasing importance over the last 15 years. In reality, the prevalence rate for anxiety disorder may be as high as, or actually be greater than, that for depressive illness

[Lenze et al., 2005b]. Anxiety as a disorder has many different subtypes, nevertheless the majority of elderly persons with a diagnosis of anxiety are actually suffering from Generalized Anxiety Disorder (GAD) and this chapter, when referring to Late-Life Anxiety Disorder, is actually referring to the onset of GAD Late-Life Anxiety. A consequence of the onset of anxiety in late-life, whether its presence was diagnosed in persons living in the community or in those admitted to hospital, is it may result in difficulties to implement treatment and rehabilitation programs for the affected elderly [Andreescu et al., 2007]. In addition, the problem of treating anxiety in the elderly is often complicated by the presence of concomitant depression, which in itself is a major factor for co-morbidity for development of anxiety.

Both depression and anxiety are two very common mood disorders in the elderly and there exist a complex interactions between the two [Harwood, Barker, Ownby & Duara, 2000; Hunt, Slade & Andrews, 2004; Williams, Peeters, & Zautra, 2004]. Depression may present with similar symptoms to anxiety and, conversely, anxiety presents with symptoms very similar to depression. The end-result is that differentiating between the two mood disorders is often extremely difficult [Krasucki, Howard, Mann, 1998; Small, 1997]. In the past many authors claimed that based on the hierarchal system, the presence of depression overrides the necessity to diagnose and treat anxiety [Beekman et al., 1998] and accordingly there is no need to relate to the anxious symptoms. However, others [Sinoff, Ore, Zlotogrosky, Tamir, 1999; Flint & Rifat, 1997] noted that many of the non-responders to treatment for depression were suffering from co-morbid anxiety and failing to relate to the anxiety component resulted in reduced or non-compliance to medication-taking in persons with concomitant depression.

This chapter will describe the onset of late-life anxiety disorder, the definition of anxiety disorder relating particularly to the problem in the elderly, the means of diagnosing the disorder relating especially to the difficulties in the elderly, and finally interaction with depression.

Anxiety Disorder in Late-Life

Anxiety has been reported to be highly prevalent in the elderly but with highly variable rates. Researchers in epidemiological studies have shown that the rates range from 5% to 20% in the elderly [The disorder is common with a prevalence rate of about 10 - 20% in the elderly population (Kvall, Laake, Engedal, 2001; Lydiard, & Brawman-Mintzer, 1998; Schuurmans et al., 2005]. Beekman and colleagues (1998) reported in the Longitudinal Aging Study of Amsterdam that 10.2% of those over 65 years had an anxiety disorder and the rates increased to 13.9% in those between the ages of 65-74. Manela and colleagues reported in their study from London that 15% of the 774 elderly subjects were diagnosed as suffering from an anxiety disorder [Manela, Katona, Livingston, 1996]. Mehta and colleagues [2003], who studied over 3,000 community-dwelling elderly between ages of 70-79, found that almost 20% of the sample had some anxiety symptoms, independent of depressive symptomatology, though, as to be expected, there was a high concurrence of depression and anxiety symptoms. Kvaal and colleagues [2001] studied 98 geriatric in-patients and compared them to 68 healthy elderly home-dwelling controls and reported that over 40% of geriatric in-patients had a diagnosis of anxiety compared to only 1% of the controls. Sadavoy and LeClair [1997] related to this problem of highly variable rates of prevalence of reported anxiety in the elderly and concluded that the major reason for such different rates may be related to the fact that anxiety disorder in the elderly is often butoftenunder-recognized and under-diagnosed. One reason for this misdiagnosis may be that It has been reported that elderly persons may not actually meet the full requirements for diagnosis of anxiety disorder and therefore are under-diagnosed with the disorder on the other hand they may still experience enough anxiety symptoms that disrupt their lives [Kogan, Edelstein, & McKee, 2000]. Other reasons may be (gary: continue sentence here)Another reason is that in the elderly there exists a high rate of physical illness with accompanying somatic complaints, and, since anxiety often presents in the elderly with somatic symptoms, the somatic symptoms may be interpreted as being part of some physical illness rather than actually relating to them as part of an anxiety disorder [Sinoff et al., 1999]. In fact, it has been reported that the elderly person has a delay of about 10 years before actually receiving medical help for his anxiety disorder [Hunt, Slade & Andrews, 2004].

The reality that anxiety in the elderly may not actually meet the full requirements for the diagnosis of anxiety disorder still does not deter from the importance to relate to the symptomatology in the elderly. As mentioned above, the elderly may still experience It has been reported thatenough anxious symptoms that disrupt their routine and activities in daily living [Hunt, Slade & Andrews, 2004; Kogan, Edelstein, & McKee, 2000]. Other reasons may be (gary: continue sentence here) This becomes important when one realizes the fact that anxiety symptomatology is very widespread in the elderly. Forsell and Winblad [1998] reported that amongst the 966 participants in the Kungsholmen Project in Stockholm Sweden, 24.4% had feelings of anxiety and 15% of these persons reported that the symptoms interfered with their Activities of Daily Living in some way. Strengthen this findings were the results from Kvall and colleagues [2001] who reported that amongst the 98 geriatric in-patients in their study, 43% had anxiety symptoms at a level to be clinically significant.

It has been disputed that the elderly, with their high rates of physical illness, have high rates of accompanying somatic complaints and since anxiety often presents in this population group with somatic symptoms, these may be interpreted as being part of some physical illness rather than actually relating to the anxiety [Sinoff et al., 1999]. The end result is that anxiety in the elderly is often missed by the treating physician since the physician is unable to differentiate between the presenting somatic symptoms such as generalized aches and pains, abdominal discomfort, or even chest pain from a medical illness [Lenze et al., 2000; Meeks, Woodruff-Borden & Depp, 2002]. Kessler and colleagues [2002] stated that up to half of those, suffering from anxiety, in fact were missed by the primary physician, partly related to the absence of relating to somatic complaints as the presenting symptom of anxiety in the old person. However, it should be borne in mind that the opposite is also true in that anxiety may mask a serious medical problem resulting in a mislabeling of a person with the medical disease as suffering from an anxiety disorder [Kogan et al., 2000] (Table 1).

The art of medicine is the ability of the clinician to relate to each problem separately and especially being able to differentiate and correctly diagnosis anxiety in the presence of medical conditions.

Table 1. Some diseases associated with anxious symptomatology.

Cardiovascular System:	Myocardial Infarction Congestive Heart Failure
Endocrine System:	Hypoglycemia Thyroid Disease
Neurological System:	Central Nervous System infection Central Nervous System masses Delirium
Hematological System:	Anemia
Immunological System:	Systemic Lupus Erythematosis
Pulmonary System:	Pneumonia Chronic Obstructive Pulmonary Disease Hypoxia
Miscellaneous	High/Low Fever Electrolyte disturbances
Dietary Problems:	Caffeine abuse Vitamin B12 Deficiency
Drug-Related	Withdrawal syndromes (Alcohol) Sedatives

Definition of Anxiety Disorder

In the field of psychiatric medicine, defining a mental disorder usually relies on the use of standardized international classification systems for the definition. In the world today there are two main systems used on both sides of the Atlantic, either the *Diagnostic and Statistical Manual of Mental Disorders* (DSM), which is used extensively in Northern American and is published by the American Psychiatric Association, or the *International Statistical Classification of Diseases and Related Health Problems* (ICD), which is used extensively in Europe and is published by the World Health Organization in Switzerland.

According to the 4th Edition of the DSM (DSM-IV), anxiety is defined as a disturbance of excessive worry occurring for most hours of the day for at least six months. There is considerable difficulty to control these feelings and the end result of the presence of this disorder is a disturbance in function on multi-levels: personal, family, social and work. Obviously the anxiety should not be related to substance abuse or another mental disorder. In addition, for the definition of anxiety disorder, a disturbance in at least three of the following areas is required: feeling restlessness, feeling tense or wound-up, tiring easily, having trouble concentrating, suffering from attacks of irritability, a significant increase in muscle tension with concomitant somatic complaints, or trouble with sleeping [APA, 1994].

In the ICD-10, the criteria are slightly different. The sufferer must have symptoms of anxiety, unrelated to a particular environment, which occurs most days during the last few weeks or even months. These symptoms should usually involve elements of: (a) apprehension (worries about future misfortunes, feeling "on edge", difficulty in concentrating), (b) motor tension (restless fidgeting, tension headaches, trembling, inability to relax); and (c) autonomic over-activity (lightheadedness, sweating, tachycardia or tachypnea, epigastric discomfort, dizziness, dry mouth) [WHO, 1993].

The essential feature is anxiety, which is generalized and persistent, but not restricted to, or even strongly predominating in, any particular environmental circumstances (i.e. it is "free-floating"). As in depression, somatic symptoms have been shown to be predominant in the elderly with an anxiety disorder and this interferes with the diagnosing the presence of an anxiety disorder [Epstein, Quill, McWhinney, 1999; Joormann & Stöber, 1999; Lenze et al., 2005; Papassotiropoulos & Heun, 1999]. The dominant symptoms are highly variable, but somatic complaints of continuous feelings of nervousness, trembling, muscular tension, sweating, lightheadedness, palpitations, dizziness, and epigastric discomfort are common. Fears that the sufferer will shortly become ill or have an accident are often expressed, together with a variety of other worries and forebodings. Anxiety disorder is more common in women, and often related to chronic environmental or life-course stresses. Its course is variable and tends to fluctuate, but is usually chronic in nature. It should be emphasized that the transient appearance of accompanying depressive symptoms does not rule out anxiety disorder as a main diagnosis.

Diagnosing Late-Life Anxiety Disorder in the Elderly

Similarly to depression, several screening instruments were developed and validated for the detection of anxiety, but none specifically for the elderly [Kogan et al., 2000]. The instruments used for the detection of anxiety range from analog rating scales such as a visual analog scale, observer-rated scales such as the Hamilton Anxiety Scale or Clinical Anxiety Scale, to self-rating scales such as the Hospital Anxiety and Depression Scale. This section is unable to relate in depth to all instruments developed but will relate to a few widely used instruments for the detection of anxiety disorder and to the development of instruments specific for the elderly. Hamilton's Rating Scale for Anxiety (HAM-A) [1959] was developed as an observer-rated scale and included fourteen items scored on a five-point scale examining anxious mood, tension, fears, insomnia, intellect, depressed mood, somatic muscular problems, somatic sensory problems and cardiovascular problems. The instrument is scored with a minimum score of 0 to a maximum score of 64 but no cut-off point has been stated to help in the diagnosis of anxiety but rather as an instrument for follow-up for detection of improvement under treatment. Snaith and colleagues [1982] in the development of their instrument, the Clinical Anxiety Scale (CAS), felt that there was a need to relate only to the anxiety and not include areas such as intellectual disabilities or depression and accordingly developed their observer-rated scale CAS with seven items examining psychic tension, ability to relax (muscular tension), startle response (hyperarousability), worrying, apprehension, restlessness and panic attacks. The items were scored on a scale from 0 to 4 giving a minimum score of 0 and a maximum score of 28. Here they used a ranging cut-off point with a score of less than 5 as being normal, 5-10 as being mildly anxious, 11-16 as being moderately anxious and 17 or more as being severely anxious. Zigmond together with Snaith [1983] felt the need to develop an instrument specifically for use in a general hospital setting to diagnose anxiety in in-patients, the Hospital Anxiety and Depression Scale (HADS), with subsections for detection of anxiety or depression. They ensured that the questions selected were such that none were related to symptoms of physical disease. The HADS-A subsection examining anxiety has seven questions investigating psychic tension, fears, worry, psychomotor agitation, panic attacks, ability to relax and somatic discomfort. Each question scored in a four-point scale from 0 to 3, so that a maximum score of 21 is obtainable. A score of 7 or less is normal, 8-10 borderline results and 11 or greater as positive score.

There have been reports that there is no suitable instrument for the detection of anxiety in the elderly [Neal & Baldwin, 1994] and even the widely employed Hospital Anxiety and Depression Scale has been criticized for use in geriatric medical inpatients [Davies, Burn, McKenzie, Brothwell, & Wattis, 1993]. In light of this problem, the Short Anxiety Screening Test (SAST) (a 10 item interviewer-assisted questionnaire) was developed to detect the presence of anxiety in the elderly, whether patients are admitted to hospital or in the community [Sinoff et al., 1999].

Table 2. Sinoff's Short Anxiety Screening Test (SAST)

Questions	Rarely or never	Sometimes	Often	Always	Points
1. Do you feel keyed up, on edge?	1	2	3	4	
2. Do you feel that something terrible is going to happen?	1	2	3	4	
3. Are you worrying about your present state?	1	2	3	4	
4. Do you feel you have control of your life?	4	3	2	1	
5. Can you relax?	4	3	2	1	
6. Do you suffer from back pain, neck pain and headache?	1	2	3	4	
7. Do you sweat a lot or suffer from palpitations?	1	2	3	4	
8. Have you been irritable?	1	2	3	4	
9. Do you sleep well?	4	3	2	1	
10. Do you suffer from dizziness or faintness?	1	2	3	4	

Key: Score ≥ 24 = positive test result Score 22-23= Borderline test results.

The concept in developing the SAST instrument was based on the fact there was an absence of instruments for diagnosing anxiety in the elderly and also to include psychic and especially somatic complaints. In many instruments, somatic complaints were often deliberately removed in other test [Goldberg, Bridges, Duncan-Jones & Grayson, 1988; Zigmond & Snaith, 1983], an omission which is reported to be a mistake, since elderly often present with major somatic complaints as a manifestation of their anxiety [Sinoff et al., 1999].

The SAST, which takes about 10 minutes to execute, includes 10 questions rated from 1 to 4 and each question has frequency choices of never or seldom, some of the time, good part of the time, or most of the time. Most of the questions are in a positive linear direction but there are some questions with a negative direction. A score of greater or equal to 24 out of a total score of 40 is regarded as positive for the presence of an anxiety disorder. The instrument conforms to the criteria for anxiety disorder set out by the DSM-IV (APA, 1994) and includes questions about vigilance ("Do you feel keyed up, on edge?"), premonition ("Do you feel that something terrible is going to happen?"), worry ("Are you worrying about your present state?"), control ("Do you feel that you have control of your life?"), tension (" Can you relax?", "Have you been irritable?"), somatic complaints ("Do you suffer from back pain, neck pain and headaches?", "Do you sweat a lot or suffer from palpitations?", " Do you suffer from dizziness or faintness?"), and sleep problems ("Do you sleep well?"). The instrument has a sensitivity of 75% and specificity of 79% with a Cronbach alpha value of 0.70.

The absence of instruments specific for the detection of anxiety in the elderly also resulted in the development of another instrument, the Geriatric Anxiety Inventory (GAI) [Pachana, Byrne, Siddle, Koloski, Harley & Arnold, 2007]. This instrument consists of twenty dichotomous response items. The authors found in their validity study that the GAI has a reported sensitivity of 75% and specificity of 84% together with a high internal consistency with Cronbach's alpha of 0.91 [Pachana et al., 2007]. There is some debate with regard to the use of instruments using dichotomous responses compared to rating scales. This was emphasized by Zigmond and Snaith [1983] in the development of their Hospital Anxiety and Depression Scale, who stated that a rating scale is more in accord with the reality for the elderly.

Interaction Between Anxiety and Depression

As stated in the introduction, anxiety is also highly associated with depression. The literature abounds with reports on the co-morbidity between depression and anxiety [Forsell & Winblad, 1998; Gottfries, 1998; Harwood, Barker, Ownby, Duara, 2000; Hunt, Slade & Andrews, 2004; Joormann and Stöber, 1999; Kogan et al., 2000; Lydiard and Brawman-Mintzer, 1998; Paterniti, Dufouil, Bisserbe & Alpérovitch, 1999; Williams, Peeters & Zautra, 2004]. In fact in the Late-Life Mood Disorder Study, Lenze and coworkers [2000] reported that amongst their 182 elderly depressed subjects, 23% had current co-morbid anxiety disorder. In the study by Mehta and colleagues [2003] of three thousand and forty-one participants, 12.3% were diagnosed as suffering from depression and 43% of these patients had co-current anxiety. Felker and coworkers [Felker et al., 2003] concluded in their study of three hundred and forty two subjects in the VA (Veterans Affairs) Primary Care Trial in the USA, that as in the findings of other studies, patients with depression were significantly more impaired when there was the presence of co-morbid anxiety symptoms. The association between the two mood disorders may take several different forms: depression with anxiety symptoms, anxiety with depressive symptoms or as a combination [Lydiard and Brawman-Mintzer, 1998]. There, therefore, exists a bi-directional diagnostic interchange between these two mood disorders, since those with anxiety may progress to depression and the opposite is also true in that those with depression may progress to develop anxiety [Forsell, 2000; Krasucki, Howard, Mann, 1998]. The importance of this is that in the past, the presence of anxiety was often missed or even worse ignored because of the DSM hierarchical exclusion rule whereby in the presence of depression, there was no need to relate to anxiety [Lenze et al., 2000]. In fact, it has been emphasized that although there is a large overlap between anxiety and depression, there is a need to make independent diagnoses as we are actually relating as two distinct constructs with overlapping features [Endler, Macrodimitris & Kocovski, 2003; Forsell and Winblad, 1998). The interaction between the two mood disorders has been termed "anxious depression" [Lydiard & Brawman-Mintzer, 1998] and the importance to relate to this state is that patients with anxious depression are less likely to respond to acute treatment [Flint & Rifat, 1997].

On a historical perspective, in the turn of the last century, Emile Kraepelin defined depression as two types: anxious or helplessness. Later Sigmund Freud addressed anxiety as a separate entity and it was felt that there existed a continuum between anxiety and depression. Nevertheless by the seventies, investigators were differentiating between anxiety and depression on the basis of symptom clusters and regarding each as a separate entity. Yet during the eighties and nineties once again it was regarded that since there is high concomitant co-morbidity and there is possibly some common pathway, then there is no need to relate to anxiety [Levine, Cole, Chenpagga & Gershon, 2001]. This theoretical model was confirmed in the findings from the study by Wittchen and colleagues which showed that anxiety is usually the primary disorder and often followed by secondary depression rather than the opposite [Wittchen, Kessler, Pfister & Leib, 2000].

However on a normal day-to-day basis in clinical setting, there is a need to identify coexisting anxiety in the presence of depression and vice versa, since each affective disorder interferes with the treatment plan of the other [Sinoff et al., 2002]. Sinoff and colleagues reported that since the treatment for depression may have a prolonged time for onset of effect, the patient may actually cease treatment because of feeling "anxious" that there is no improvement and relief from his depressive symptoms [Sinoff et al., 1999]. If by relating to and diagnosing the presence of an anxiety disorder, then early concomitant treatment directed towards the anxiety, may actually result in higher compliance for treatment for the depressive disorder. In fact often the initial positive reaction to treatment of anti-depressants is actually related to the anxiolytic effect of the anti-depressants themselves.

Conclusion

Anxiety has been now recognized as a major mood disorder in the elderly and as stated above it may actually have a prevalence rate greater than that for depression. The problem in the elderly has been to define anxiety in late-life. Some authors feel that the inclusions of somatic symptoms unfairly diagnose anxiety in patients with a medical illness since obviously a person with a medical illness will have somatic symptoms. On the other hand, others feel that not relating to somatic symptoms especially in the elderly is a major drawback in diagnosing an anxiety disorder since the elderly usually present with somatic complaints as an expression of their mood problems, whether it be depression or anxiety [Joormann & Stobe, 1999; Lenze et al., 2005; Sinoff et al., 1999]. To the belief of this author, there exists high significance to use somatic symptoms as part of the symptoms in the diagnosing of anxiety in late-life thereby ensuring the diagnosis by means of the DSM-IV criteria. The problem arises in the means of diagnosing the disorder. Many instruments have been developed over the years for diagnosing anxiety, although only a few have been specifically designed for diagnosing anxiety in the elderly. The dilemma arises whether to use a dichotomous scale or a rating scale; a visual analogue scale, an observer-rated scale, self-rating scale or a structure interview schedule or to rely purely on clinical assessment by a psychiatrist. The advantage of the SAST instrument developed by this author is that it was also validated to detect anxiety even in the presence of depression. Unfortunately, routine administration of instruments has been shown not to influence untrained clinicians in the decision-making process and translate into improved management of mood disorders [Gilbody, O'House & Sheldon, 2001].

Recently, Lenze and Wetherell [2008] emphasized the importance of detecting and relating to Late-Life Anxiety Disorder since it is associated with functional impairment, poorer quality of life and adverse long-term consequences such as cognitive decline. This chapter has not dealt at all with the different approaches to treatment of anxiety in the elderly, both psychological and pharmacological, which in themselves are major hurdles that faces the physician in the daily routine of clinical work with the elderly. There is a need however to relate to the interaction between late-life anxiety and cognition which will be discussed in the next chapter.

REFERENCES

American Psychiatric Association (APA). (1994). *Diagnostic and Statistical Manual of Mental Disorders* (Fourth Edition). Washington, D.C.: American Psychiatric Association.

Andreescu, C., Lenze, E.J., Dev, M.A., Begley, H.E., Mulsant, B.H., Dombrovski, A.Y., Pollock, B.G., Stack, J., Miller, M.D., & Reynolds, C.F. (2007). Effect of comorbid anxiety on treatment response and relapse risk in late-life depression: Controlled study. *British Journal of Psychiatry, 190,* 344-349.

Beekman, A.T.F., Bremmer, M.A., Deeg, D.J.H., van Balkom, A.J.L.M., Smit, J.H., De Beurs, E., van Dyck, R., & van Tilburg, W. (1998). Anxiety disorders in later life: A report from the longitudinal aging study Amsterdam. *International Journal of Geriatric Psychiatry, 13,* 717-726.

Davies, K.N., Burn, W.K., McKenzie, F.R., Brothwell, J.A., & Wattis, J.P. (1993). Evaluation of the hospital anxiety and depression scale as a screening instrument in geriatric medical inpatients. *International Journal of Geriatric Psychiatry,8* (2), 165-169

Endler, N.S., Macrodimitris, S.D., & Kocovski, N.L. (2003). Anxiety and depression: Congruent, separate, or both? *Journal of Applied Biobehavioral Research, 8,* 42-60.

Epstein, R.M., Quill, T.E., & McWhinney, I.R. (1999). Somatization reconsidered. Incorporating the patient's experience of illness. *Archives of Internal Medicine, 159,* 215-222.

Felker, B.L., Hedrick, S.C., Chaney, E.F., Liu, C.F., Heagerty, P., Caples, H., Lin, P., & Katon, W. 2003. Identifying depressed patients with a high risk of comorbid anxiety in primary care. *Prim Care Companion Journal of Clinical Psychiatry,5,* 104-110.

Forsell, Y. (2000). Predictors for depression, anxiety and psychotic symptoms in a very elderly population: Data from a 3-year follow-up study. *Social Psychiatry and Psychiatry Epidemiology, 35,*259-263.

Forsell, Y., & Winblad, B. (1998). Feelings of anxiety and associated variables in a very elderly population. *International Journal of Geriatric Psychiatry, 13,* 454–458.

Gilbody, S.M., O-House, A., & Sheldon, T.A. (2001). Routinely administered questionnaires for depression and anxiety: Systematic review. *British Medical Journal, 322,* 406-409.

Goldberg, D., Bridges, K., Duncan-Jones, P., & Grayson, D. (1988). Detecting anxiety and depression in general medical setting. *British Medical Journal, 297*, 897-898.

Gottfries, C.G. (1998). Is there a difference between elderly and younger patients with regard to the symptomatology and aetiology of depression? *International Clinical Psychopharmacology, 13*(suppl 5), S13–S18.

Hamilton, M. (1959). The assessment of anxiety states by rating. *British Journal of Medical Psychology, 32,*50-55.

Harwood, D.G., Barker, W.W., Ownby, R.L., & Duara, R. (2000). Relationship of behavioral and psychological symptoms to cognitive impairment and functional status in Alzheimer's disease. *International Journal of Geriatric Psychiatry, 15,* 393-400.

Hunt, C., Slade, T., & Andrews, G. (2004). Generalized Anxiety Disorder and major depressive disorder comorbidity in the National Survey of Mental Health and Well-Being. *Depression and Anxiety, 20*(1), 23-31.

Joormann, J., & Stöber, J. (1999). Somatic symptoms of Generalized Anxiety Disorder from the DSM-IV: Associations with pathological worry and depression symptoms in a nonclinical sample. *Journal of Anxiety Disorder, 13* (5), 491–503.

Kessler, D., Bennewith, O., Lewis, G., & Sharp, D. (2002). Detection of depression and anxiety in primary care: Follow-up study. *British Medical Journal, 325,*1016-1017.

Kogan, J.N., Edelstein, B.A., & McKee, D.R. (2000). Assessment of anxiety in older adults: Current status. *Journal of Anxiety Disorder, 14*(2), 109–132.

Krasucki, C., Howard, R., & Mann, A. (1998). The relationship between anxiety disorders and age. *International Journal of Geriatric Psychiatry, 13,* 79–99.

Kvaal, K., Laake, K., & Engedal, K. (2001). Psychometric properties of the state part of the Spielberger state-trait anxiety inventory (STAI) in geriatric patients. *International Journal of Geriatric Psychiatry, 16* (10), 980-986.

Kvall, K., Macijauskiene, J., Engedal, K., & Laake, K. (2001). High prevalence of anxiety symptoms in hospitalized geriatric patients. *International Journal of Geriatric Psychiatry, 16*, 690-693.

Lenze, E.J., Mulsant, B.H., Mohlman, J., Shear, M.K., Dew, M.A., Schulz, R., Miller, M.D., Tracey, B., & Reynolds III, C.F. (2005). Generalized anxiety disorder in late life: lifetime course and comorbidity with major depressive disorder. *American Journal of Geriatric Psychiatry, 13*(1), 77-80.

Lenze, E.J., Mulsant, B.H., Shear, M.K., Schulberg, H.C., Dew, M.A., Begley, A.E., Pollock, B.G., & Reynolds III, C.F. (2000). Comorbid anxiety disorders in depressed elderly patients. *American Journal of Psychiatry, 157*(5), 722–728.

Lenze, E.J., & Wetherell, J.L. (2008). Bringing the bedside to the bench, and then to the community: a prospectus for intervention research in late-life anxiety disorders. *International Journal of the Geriatric Psychiatry, 24* (1), 1-14.

Levine, J., Cole, D.P., Chengapp, K.N.R., & Gershon, S. (2001). Anxiety disorders and major depression, together or apart. *Depression and Anxiety, 14*, 94-104.

Lydiard, R.B., & Brawman-Mintzer, O. (1998). Anxious depression. *Journal of Clinical Psychiatry,* 59(supplement 18), 10–17.

Manela, M., Katona, C., & Livingston, G. (1996). How common are the anxiety disorders in old age? *International Journal of Geriatric Psychiatry, 11*,65–70.

Meeks, S., Woodruff-Borden, J., & Depp, C.A. (2003). Structural differentiation of self-reported depression and anxiety in late-life. *Journal of Anxiety Disorders, 17* (6), 627-646.

Mehta, K.M., Simonsick, E.M., Penninx, B.W.J.H., Schulz, R., Rubin, S.M., Satterfield, S., & Yaffe, K. (2003). Prevalence and correlates of anxiety symptoms in well-functioning older adults: Findings from the Healthy Aging and Body Composition Study. *Journal of the American Geriatrics Society, 51,* 499-504.

Neal, R.M., & Baldwin, R.C. (1994). Screening for anxiety and depression in elderly medical outpatients. *Age and Ageing, 23*, 462-464.

Pachana, N.A., Byrne, G.J., Siddle, H., Koloski, N., Harley, E., & Arnold, E. (2007). Development and validation of the Geriatric Anxiety Inventory. *International Psychogeriatrics, 19* (1), 103-114.

Papassotiropoulos, A., & Heun, R. (1999). Detection of subthreshold depression and subthreshold anxiety in the elderly. *International Journal of Geriatric Psychiatry, 14,*643–650.

Paterniti, S., Dufouil, C., Bisserbe, J.C., Alpérovitch, A. (1999). Anxiety, depression, psychotropic drug use and cognitive impairment. *Psychological Medicine, 29,* 421-428.

Sadavoy, J., & LeClair, J.K. (1997). Treatment of anxiety disorders in late life. *Canadian Journal of Psychiatry, 42*(Suppl 1), 28S–34S.

Schuurmans, J., Comijs, H.C., Beekman, A.T., de Beurs, E., Deeg, D.J., Emmelkamp, P.M., & van Dyck, R. (2005). The outcome of anxiety disorders in older people at 6-year follow-up: results from the Longitudinal Aging Study Amsterdam. *Acta Psychiatry Scandanavia, 111*(6), 420-428.

Sinoff, G., Ore, L., Zlotogorsky, D., & Tamir, A. (1999). Short anxiety screening test – a brief instrument for detecting anxiety in the elderly. *International Journal of Geriatric Psychiatry, 14*(12), 1062–1071.

Sinoff, G., Ore, L., Zlotogorsky, D., & Tamir, A. (2002). Does the presence of anxiety affect the validity of a screening test for depression in the elderly? *International Journal of Geriatric Psychiatry, 17*(4), 309-314.

Small, G.W. (1997). Recognizing and treating anxiety in the elderly. *Journal of Clinical Psychiatry, 58*(suppl 3), 41-47.

Snaith, R.P., Baugh, S.J., Clayden, A.D., Husain, A., & Sipple, M.A. (1982). The Clinical Anxiety Scale: An instrument derived from the Hamilton Anxiety Scale. *British Journal of Psychiatry,141*, 518-523.

Williams, J., Peeters, F., & Zautra, A. (2004). Differential affect structure in depressive and anxiety disorders. *Anxiety, Stress and Coping, 17*(4), 321-330.

Wittchen, H.U., Kessler, K.C., Pfister, H., & Leib, M. (2000). Why do people with anxiety disorders become depressed? A prospective-longitudinal community study. *Acta Psychiatry Scandanavia Supplement* (406),14-23.

World Health Organization (WHO). (1993). *The ICD-10. Classification of Mental and Behavioural Disorders. Diagnostic Criteria for Research.* Geneva, Switzerland: World Health Organization.

Zigmond, A.S., & Snaith, R.P. (1983). The hospital anxiety and depression scale. *Acta Psychiatry Scandanavia, 67*(6), 361-370.

In: Psychiatric Research Trends: Dreams and Geriatric Psychiatry ISBN 978-1-60741-760-6
Editors: Daniella M. Montez, pp.79-99

Chapter 5

LATE-LIFE ANXIETY AND MILD COGNITIVE IMPAIRMENT

Gary Sinoff
Director, Cognitive Clinic, Department of Geriatrics, Carmel Medical Center, Haifa, Israel and
Department of Gerontology, University of Haifa, Mt.Carmel, Haifa, Israel

ABSTRACT

Cognitive decline has become a major burden to society, so if one could delay the decline by initiating treatment as early as possible, the savings for both the individual and society would be significant. The importance of relating to Mild Cognitive Impairment concerns the high annual conversion rates of up to 30% for this disorder. Thus, the importance of finding the predictors for further cognitive decline is of the highest priority. Researchers have proposed the use of neuroimaging, biomarkers, use of EEG brain wave patterns, neuropsychological testing or a combination of them. Amongst the neuropsychological clinical entities examined have been the mood disorders depression and anxiety. Depression has been reported to be a predictor for future cognitive decline, but with regard to anxiety, the question is debatable. In some studies of elderly with memory problems, the presence of anxiety was highly predictive of future cognitive decline. However in studies with MCI cohorts, though anxiety is found in up to 40% of MCI sufferers, it was found not to be a predictor. A possible theoretical explanation is that elderly turning for an assessment are at Braak's stage I/II and in those diagnosed with MCI, are at Braak's stage III/IV. At the earlier stages (stage I/II), flow of information via the entorhinal cortex to the hippocampus is impaired resulting in hyperactivity of the alternate pathway of the amygdala, which explains the high prevalence of anxiety. However, by the time a person turns to a specialized cognitive clinic and is diagnosed with amnestic-MCI (stage III /IV) flow via the alternative pathway of the amygdala though present, is now partially impaired. After conversion to dementia (stage V), only a few were still with anxiety since now the pathway to the amygdala was also impaired. In conclusion, anxiety is prominent in persons with amnestic MCI, but this did not predict future cognitive decline, perhaps since persons with MCI turning for cognitive assessment, probably have early onset of dementia. There does however seem to be a trend that those with anxiety and MCI do tend to develop cognitive decline at slight higher rates.

INTRODUCTION

In the previous chapter, late-life anxiety disorder was described in relation to the description and definition of the disorder, the means of diagnosing the disorder, and finally its interaction with depression. In this chapter, the interaction between anxiety and cognitive decline will be discussed. With the increase over the last few decades in the percentage of elderly in the general population, cognitive decline in the aged has become a major burden for health care services in the present millennium. For the young elderly (under 70 years) the prevalence rate for dementia is around 10% but this increases four-fold to 40% by the age of 85 years [Petersen, Stevens, Ganguli, Tangalos, Cummings and DeKosky, 2001]. As a consequence, society has found its resources strained and with too few places in institutions for the demented elderly. If one is able to delay the cognitive decline by even a few months, then the savings financially, both on a national and personal level, would be significant [DeKosky, 2003; Sadik and Wilcock, 2003]. In fact in 2003 the cost in USA for the treatment of Alzheimer's disease was reported to be close to $90 billion [Karlawish, Casarett, James, Tenhave, Clark and Asch, 2003]. Since cognitive decline develops over an extended period of time and because of new treatment modalities on the market, the importance of identifying predictors of future cognitive decline has also become relevant [Collie and Maruff, 2000; DeKosky and Marek, 2003; Visser, Verhey, Ponds, Cruts, Van Broeckhoven and Jolles, 2000]. Amongst the predictors has been claimed the presence of mood disorders, depression and probably anxiety.

Once a person is diagnosed with dementia, irrespective of the type, the efficacy of treatment, usually cholinesterase inhibitors, decreases with the disease's progression. Starting treatment in the early stages of the disease has been found to decrease care-giver burden and even delay institutionalization for up to a year [Lanctôt et al., 2003]. The importance of relating to the early stages of cognitive decline, termed Mild Cognitive Impairment (MCI), is the evidence of high annual conversion rates to dementia (10-20% per year) [Boyle, Wilson, Aggarwal, Tang and Bennett, 2006; Petersen, Smith, Waring, Ivnik, Tangalso and Kokmen, 1999; Waite, Broe, Grayson and Creasey, 2001].

In a previous study by this author, it was found that some of those requesting a consultation in a geriatric community assessment unit clinic were suffering from anxiety, and usually, accompanied by concomitant memory loss [Sinoff and Werner, 2003]. In the final analysis it was revealed that in those with anxiety had a relative risk of 3.96 for developing future cognitive decline as defined by a change of more than 2 points on the Mini-Mental State Examination, emphasizing the need to relate, also, to the interaction between anxiety and cognitive impairment.

This chapter will relate to Mild Cognitive Impairment (MCI) – its clinical manifestation and diagnosis, the possible predictors of future cognitive decline in MCI, interaction between anxiety and Mild Cognitive Impairment, and, finally, a proposed model of MCI with regard to the presence of anxiety based on findings from this author's previous study and findings from a recent unpublished study by this author.

MILD COGNITIVE IMPAIRMENT - ITS CLINICAL MANIFESTATION AND DIAGNOSIS

In the 1990s, Flicker and colleagues [1991] from New York Medical Center, and Petersen and his colleagues from Mayo Clinic [1994] concurrently decided on the term Mild Cognitive Impairment (MCI). Petersen's group defined it as a complaint of memory loss reported by the patient, by the family or by his physician without evidence of dementia as defined by *Diagnostic and Statistical Manual of Mental Disorders* 4th Edition (DSM-IV) [APA 1994]; with normal performance in activities of daily living and normal global cognitive function, but with an objective memory loss greater than 1.5 SD on neuropsychological testing, while controlling for age and education [Petersen et al., 1999].

MCI defines a transitional state between the state of cognitive changes of normal aging and mild dementia [Chertkow, 2002; Dierckx, Engelborghs, De Raedt, De Deyn and Ponjaert-Kristoffersen, 2007; Morris, Storandt, Miller, Price, Rubin, and Berg, 2001; Petersen et al., 2001; Zaudig, 2002] and has been divided into three subtypes: amnestic-MCI, multiple domains-MCI, or single non-memory domain-MCI. The definition of Mild Cognitive Impairment includes a person's self-awareness of loss of memory, termed metamemory, which refers to the knowledge people have about their own memory problems [Pannu and Kaszniak, 2005; Ponds and Jolles, 1996]. When the elderly have a memory problem, they have no way of knowing whether they are in danger of impending cognitive decline or are experiencing a transient phenomenon. In fact, this metamemory disturbance may be the driving force behind the decision to turn to a physician for advice and is regarded as the major component of the amnestic subgroup of MCI. Palmer and colleagues [2003] reported in their study of 1435 persons aged 75-95 in the Kungsholmen cohort in Stockholm, that to diagnose MCI requires a three step process: searching for a memory complaint, assessing for global cognitive impairment and performing neuropsychological testing.

Clinically, MCI is a common disorder amongst the aged and has a prevalence rate ranging between 10-20% in the general elderly population [Di Carlo et al., 2000; Graham et al., 1997; Petersen et al., 2001; Zaudig, 2002], with rates rising with the old-elderly [Hänninen, Hallikainen, Toumainen, Vanhanen, and Soininen, 2002]. In the Sydney Older Persons Study from Australia, the rate for a preclinical syndrome including cognitive deficits was reported to be as high as 31.3% for their cohort of 537 elderly persons [Waite et al., 2001]. Manly and her colleagues [2005] reported a similar high rate of 28.3% for MCI in their study of 1315 non-demented elderly in the community in the New York area.

As mentioned above, the importance of diagnosing MCI is that people experiencing MCI have a greater risk for conversion to dementia at a later stage [Christensen, Henderson, Korten, Jorm, Jacomb and Mackinnon, 1997; Friedrich, 1999; Ritchie and Touchon, 2000; Shah, Tangalos and Petersen, 2000]. Morris and his colleagues [2001] reported that all of their 277 MCI subjects converted to dementia within 5 years. Similarly all 10 MCI subjects in the study by Hodges, Erzinçlioğlu and Patterson [2006] converted to dementia within 6 years. In the community based PAQUID study, Larrieu and colleagues [2002] reported an annual conversion rate to dementia of 8.3% per year in their 58 MCI subjects. In another population-based study from Paris, a conversion rate of 32.2% over 2 years was reported in a cohort of 90 persons with MCI [Amieva et al., 2004], that is an annual conversion rate of 16.2%. From the Canadian Study of Health and Aging, the conversion rate in 801 persons with CIND

(Cognitive Impairment Not Demented) was 47% compared to 15% in no cognitive impairment over 5 years [Tuokko et al., 2003], an annual conversion rate of 9.4%. For the Cache County Study on Memory Health and Aging, a 3-year conversion rate of 45.8% was found [Tschanz et al. 2006], an annual conversion rate of 15.2%. In the Maastricht Memory Clinic cohort, overall 30% of the 145 subjects converted to dementia within 10 years [Visser, Kestner, Jolles and Verhey, 2006]. In the study by Sinoff and Werner [2003], 30% of the 100 subjects in the community study converted to dementia within 3.2 years giving an annual conversion rate of 9.3%. Luis and colleagues (2003) reviewed the literature and emphasized the importance of diagnosing MCI because of these high conversion rates of MCI to dementia from 10-30% annually and up to 50-100% in 5-10 years.

In 2003, the International Working Group on Mild Cognitive Impairment in Stockholm arrived at a consensus for the clinical definition of MCI emphasizing that there exists evidence of cognitive decline over time which is either self-reported and/or informant reported with no evidence of dementia, but with preservation of basic activities of daily living or only minimal impairment in complex instrumental functions [Winblad et al., 2004].

Ganguli [2006] stated in her review article on the constructs of MCI that "(researchers) are studying an ill defined entity with no biomarker and no gold standard" and concluded that "(the) most pressing interest in MCI epidemiology today is identifying the characteristics that predict progression." Therefore, there exists a need to find the predictors of future conversion to dementia in persons diagnosed with MCI.

Possible Predictors of Future Cognitive Decline in MCI

When one realizes that, within a few years, 25-30% or higher of those persons with MCI will develop full-blown dementia, the need for predictors becomes of great importance [Busse, Bischkopf, Riedel-Heller and Angermeyer, 2003; Chertkow, 2002; Palmer, Berger, Monastero, Winblad, Bäckman, Fratiglioni, 2007; Petersen et al., 2001; Wahlund, Philstrand and Jönhagen, 2003].

While examining the subsets of MCI (amnestic, multi-domain and single domain) mentioned above, Petersen [2000] claimed that the amnestic type is more predictive of future dementia of Alzheimer type, and the multi-domain type for developing vascular dementia. However, Verhey's group reported in their study of 118 cognitively impaired non-demented persons that the multiple domain MCI subtype had the highest predictive accuracy [Rasquin, Lodder, Visser, Lousberg and Verhey, 2005], a finding supported by Storandt and colleagues [Storandt, Grant, Miller and Morris, 2006] who found that only 61% of their MCI subjects who converted, had reported memory deficits. In contrast, Zanetti and co-workers [2006] in their study of 31 subjects with amnestic subtype and 34 with multiple domain subtype, still found a higher conversion rate to dementia with the amnestic subtype with 35% of the subjects developing dementia compared to 26% of those with multi-domain. Busse and colleagues [2003] found that amongst their study population of 62 MCI subjects, no difference in the individual predictive value of the subtypes was found and concluded that all three subsets together are required to obtain significant predictive power for the onset of dementia. On the other hand, Alexopoulos and fellow researchers [2006] in their study of 81 subjects with MCI found that 25% of amnestic subtype, 54% of multi-domain and 37.5% of single non-memory domain converted to dementia and these findings tend to reinforce the feelings of Busse and colleagues [2003] that it is unnecessary to subtype MCI.

Knowledge about which variables are predictors of future dementia is still in debate. Since treating all those with MCI would be expensive and unfeasible, there is a pressing need to find those predictors. Some research has shown neuroimaging to be useful [DeCarli et al., 2007; Modrego, Fayed and Pina, 2005], while other research has been directed at biomarkers [Bookheimer et al., 2000; Galasko, 2001] or use of EEG brain wave patterns [Huang, Wahlund, Dierks, Julin, Winblad and Jelic, 2000]. In a review by Wolf and colleagues [2003], the authors reported that based on neuroimaging, a correct classification of MCI and normal controls was about 75% when related to hippocampal and entorhinal cortex atrophy. Modrego and colleagues [2005] reported a sensitivity of 100% and a specificity of 75% for prediction of dementia using brain magnetic resonance spectroscopy in their study on 53 persons with MCI. However, Adak and colleagues [2004] felt that use of neuroimaging alone was insufficient and reported that the use of a combination of simple clinical tests (such as the MMSE) together with MRI volumes better predicted progression to dementia in their sample of 20 subjects with MCI at baseline. Regarding biomarkers, Herukka and colleagues [2005] reported on 124 patients with an extended follow-up period that the most predictive test for dementia involved a combination of β-amyloid and phospho-τ in the CSF. Some researchers have suggested the combination of neuroimaging and biomarkers for improving the diagnosis of MCI [de Leon et al., 2006]. However, most physicians have limited access to neuroimaging and even less to biomarkers, and tend, therefore, to rely on clinical and neuropsychological predictors [Petersen et al., 2001, Tian, Bucks, Haworth and Wilcock, 2006]. The multi-center Alzheimer's Disease Cooperative Study found that neuropsychological tests in their cohort of 769 participants were accurate enough for diagnosing MCI and are sensitive enough for use in future prediction studies [Grundman et al., 2004]. In fact, Griffith and co-workers [2006] reported in their study of 49 MCI patients, that by means of various neuropsychological tests they correctly classified 81.3% of those with amnestic-MCI.

Amongst the neuropsychological clinical entities examined, depression has been investigated as a clinical predictor. Depression is common in those with memory complaints and in a study by Edwards, Lindquist and Yaffe [2004], 38.7% of their 499 subjects visiting a memory clinic had clinical depression at initial consult for memory complaints. In fact, reports in the literature noted that a mood disorder usually occurs in the very early stages of cognitive decline [Harwood, Barker, Ownby, and Duara, 2000; Lee, Potter, Wagner, Welsh-Bohmer and Steffens, 2007]. In a study of 1116 community dwelling elderly persons aged 65 years, Paterniti and colleagues [1999] found that in the community, both depression and anxiety, had an effect on cognition. However, others report that anxiety and depression occurred as a reaction to the onset of cognitive decline [Devanand et al., 1996; Jorm, Christensen, Korten, Henderson, Jacomb and Mackinnon, 1997]. Wilson and colleagues [2007] reported in the findings from the Religious Order Study that psychological distress in old age might be an early sign of the pathology of Alzheimer's disease or alternatively may modify the impact on cognitive function. They reported an inverse relationship to global cognition for anxiety (adjusted regression coefficient = -0.04) and for depression (adjusted regression coefficient = -0.12) but were unable to find a correlation with any specific neuropathology. They concluded that different novel neurodegenerative mechanisms may be involved in dementia and psychological distress. Starkstein and colleagues [2007] reported a high correlation between anxiety and depression in their 552 patients with probable dementia and this was associated with more severe cognitive deficits.

It has been shown that patient's self-perceptions of memory changes are often unrecognized by the patient's family and even the patient himself may not be aware of the extent of the cognitive deficits [Cutler and Hodgson, 1996; Derouesné, Thibault, Lagha-Pierucci, Baudouin-Madec, Ancri and Lacomblez, 1999]. This may cause a feeling of despair with a resultant disturbance of mood [Small et al., 2001], since the person has not been given confirmation of his subjective feelings of memory loss. Resulting from this, they may present with depression [Harwood et al., 2000] or with anxiety as a manifestation of their memory loss [Sinoff and Werner, 2003].

Studies showed that depression may present together with cognitive problems and may actually be the first sign of the onset of an early stage of dementia. In the MIRAGE study, 4046 individuals were investigated and an OR of 4.6 was found for developing dementia in persons with depression [Green et al., 2003]. In fact depression is very common in the pre-clinical stages of Alzheimer's Disease, i.e. at the prodromal stage of MCI [Berger, Fratiglioni, Forsell, Winblad, Bäckman., 1999; Rubin, Veiel, Kinscherf, Morris, Storandt, 2001; Wilson et al., 2002]. In the Italian Longitudinal Study, it was reported that amongst their 139 subjects with MCI, 63.3% had depressive symptoms [Solfrizzi et al., 2007]. Li, Meyer and Thornby [2001] found that 28% of all the MCI patients and 57% of MCI patients who developed dementia had depression at the onset of the study. The fact of depression in the prodromal stage as a predictor of future cognitive decline was reinforced recently in a study by Geda and colleagues [2006], who reported that in a cohort of 840 cognitively normal persons, those who developed depression, had a subsequent higher risk for developing MCI (Hazard ratio of 2.2). Crowe and colleagues [2006] reported that amongst their 55 subjects with MCI, a significant correlation was found between depression and change in cognitive function (r=0.47). They concluded that depression was a reflection of the cognitive decline rather than the opposite. In a study from Poland, it was found that 55.2% of the 105 subjects with MCI, many had depression and that there exists a significant relationship between depression and progression to dementia [Gabryelewicz et al., 2007]. Modregro and Ferrandez [2004] showed a relative risk of 2.6 for development of dementia in persons with MCI if suffering from depression. They reported 35/41 of their depressed subjects developed dementia compared to only 24/73 of their non-depressed subjects. The authors concluded that depression in patients with MCI increases the risk of developing dementia, or at least lends to a faster rate of cognitive decline. Visser and colleagues [2000] hypothesized that cognitive decline may actually not be a result of depression but rather the opposite is true, i.e. depression is a manifestation of the cognitive decline. Small and co-workers [2001] studied 66 persons with MCI and found an association between depressive symptoms and subjective memory loss but only in the presence of a genetic marker for dementia. However, they concluded that the depressive symptoms were related to the memory loss rather than the opposite. DeLuca and her co-authors [2005] actually reported that amongst their 79 elderly depressed patients, those with co-morbid anxiety showed greater memory decline on the memory subsection of the Mattis' Dementia Rating Scale. With regard to anxiety, studies are lacking. In a study of 260 elderly persons attending a memory clinic, the presence of anxiety was highly correlated with reported memory complaints and was found to influence the cognitive functioning of the older person [Derousné et al., 1999].

In summary, both anxiety and depression have been shown to occur commonly with early dementia [Flint, 1994]. A person may not be aware of his declining mental functioning but feels that something is wrong, which is accompanied by concomitant feelings of anxiety or depression [Schneider, 1996]. The question remains as to whether anxiety alone is a contributing factor to cognitive decline.

ANXIETY AND MILD COGNITIVE IMPAIRMENT

Depression and anxiety are very common in Alzheimer disease, and it has been reported that almost 90% of persons with Alzheimer's disease have one of these symptoms [Mega, Cummings, Fiorello and Gornbein, 1996]. In the LASER-AD study, it was shown that 75% of the 198 subjects with AD had a mood baseline symptom and 80% of these subjects had persistent symptoms after 6 months [Ryu, Katona, Rive and Livingston , 2005]. In a study of 100 subjects requesting geriatric assessment in the community, it was found that those with memory loss and accompanying anxiety had a relative risk of 3.96 for future cognitive decline [Sinoff and Werner, 2003]. Ownby and colleagues [2000] found that anxiety symptoms were common in patients with dementia. In fact, they found that over 60% of their 133 patients presented with anxiety symptoms. Hwang from Cummings' group at UCLA reported that 75% of the 28 subjects with MCI had neuropsychiatric symptoms compared to 89% of the 124 persons in the mild AD group and 12% of the 50 subjects in the control group [Hwang, Masterman, Ortiz, Fairbanks and Cummings, 2004]. Lyketsos et al. [2002] in their study of 138 persons with MCI, found that neuropsychiatric symptoms were prevalent in 29% of the subjects. Feldman and colleagues [2004] found that 60% of their 1,010 subjects in their MCI cohort reported neuropsychiatric symptoms, with similar rates for depression and anxiety. Clare and her colleagues in the UK [2002] reported that 41% of their 94 patients with AD had anxiety compared to only 12% had depression. These studies reinforce the reality that anxiety is a common disorder in those with cognitive impairment from those with MCI to those diagnosed with dementia, probably more prevalent than depression. In fact on examining the presence of anxiety and depression in MCI, Forsell and her co-workers at the Karolinski Institute in Stockholm [2003] established that the only psychiatric complaint present amongst the 89 patients diagnosed with MCI was anxiety. Tatsch and colleagues [2006] reported in their study of 25 persons with CIND in their community study that the most prevalent symptoms were anxiety and sleep disturbances (24% each), rather than depression. Bierman and others [2005] showed that initially mild anxiety symptoms seemed to be beneficial to cognition but ultimately severe anxiety negatively influenced cognitive performance.

Theoretical Model for Explaining the Interaction between Anxiety and Cognition

Based on the literature, one could propose a theoretical model that at the time of diagnosis of early cognitive decline i.e. at the onset of MCI, anxiety may be prominent and with time the person may develop either depression, cognitive decline or continue with anxiety and if the persons were followed-up long enough, they would eventually develop dementia.

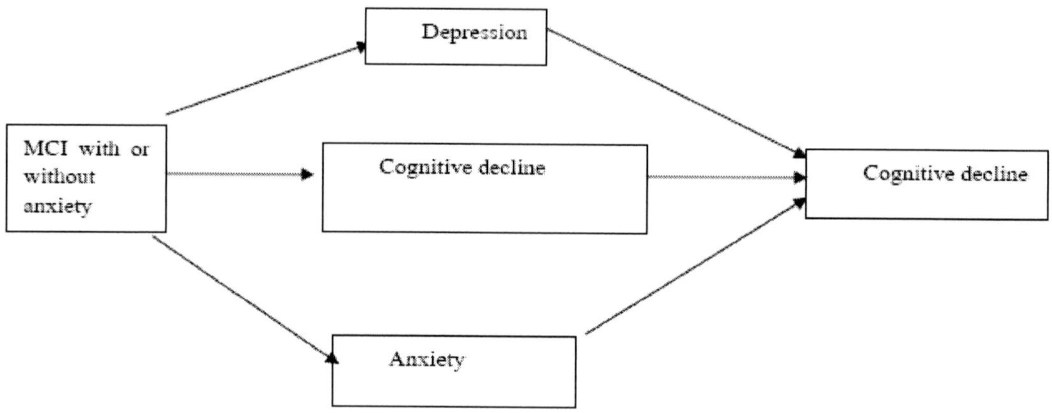

Figure 1. Theoretical model.

Conceptually, the stage of MCI is important to examine, since the process of memory loss is a long and protracted one occurring over a decade or more [Collie and Maruff, 2000; Petersen and Morris, 2005; Waite, et al., 2001]. It is probable that those turning to a memory clinic for cognitive assessment may actually be at an early stage of dementia which may explain the high conversion rates (rates of 35-30%) [Visser, Kester, Jolles and Verhey, 2006].

Interestingly in a recent unpublished study by this author [Sinoff, 2007] there was a high prevalence rate for anxiety (35%) with a lower rate for depression (13.9%). Many authors have found that amongst the neuropsychiatric syndromes associated with MCI, anxiety is very prominent, often more than depression. In the Maastricht Study in the Netherlands, it was reported that 95% of the subjects developed at least one clinically relevant neuropsychiatric problem during the course of dementia [Aalten, de Vugt, Jaspers, Jolles and Verhey, 2005] mostly anxiety and depression. Recently, Palmer and colleagues [2007] reported that anxiety was very prominent in persons with MCI, even more than depression. They concluded that persons suffering from MCI with anxiety had an increased relative risk of progression to Alzheimer's disease over 3 years compared with persons with MCI without anxiety. Similar findings by Sinoff and Werner [2003] in their community-based geriatric assessment unit study. However, in the unpublished study of this author [Sinoff, 2007] though anxiety was prevalent in persons diagnosed with MCI (36%), it was not found to be a predictor of future cognitive decline or dementia after two years.

The disparity in the findings between the author's two studies [Sinoff and Werner, 2003; Sinoff, 2007] may actually be related to a novel alternative theoretical mode. A possible neuro-anatomical explanation can be found in the model of development of Alzheimer Disease proposed by the findings of Braak, Del Tredici and Braak [2003] (See Figures 2-4).

The process of memory retention starts with the senses, which absorb information from somato-sensory inputs of hearing by the ears, sight by the eyes and feel by somatosensors. This information is relayed to the primary sensory cortex situated in the anteromedial portions of the temporal lobe, continues through to the first order sensory association area and then to the high order sensory association area. At this stage, two possible pathways exist;

information is transferred either to the amygdala and allocortex or directly to pre-frontal association area. It has been postulated that the flow of information enters both the entorhinal region and the amygdala simultaneously and then to the hippocampus. The brain regions shown to be critically important for memory are the hippocampus and the entorhinal cortex and are affected very early in individuals with MCI [Modrego et al., 2005; Stoub, deToledo-Morrell, Stabbins, Leurgans, Bennet, and Shah, 2006]. (see Figure 2).

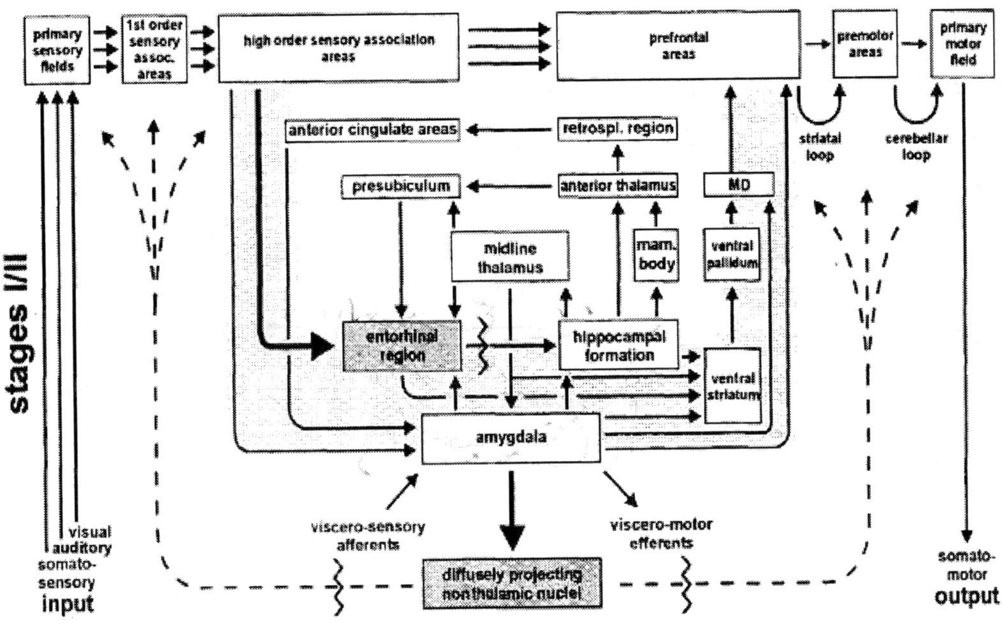

Figure 2. Model of development of interference of information transfer according to Braak and Braak Stages I/II (Reprinted with permission from Braak, Del Tredici and Braak, 2003).

At the very early stages of degenerative process, the neuroanatomical pathological findings of neurofibrillary degeneration are in the transentorhinal area, Braak Stage 1 [Braak, Del Tredici and Braak, 2003] and this causes a slight break in transferring afferent information from the sensory area into the hippocampus [Stoub et al., 2006]. In fact, these changes of neurofibillary tangles in the entorhinal and transentorhinal cortices have been reported in persons around the age of 60 years, the age when often persons start to complain about subjective memory loss [Guillozet, Weintraub, Mash and Mesulam, 2003]. By stage II the degenerative process has progressed and involves the whole entorhinal area region.

From the neuro-anatomical model, what is occurring is that the amygdala is still receiving information resulting in hypertrophy of the amygdala, but the hippocampus is being denied the flow of unobstructed information and starts to atrophy. It is known by radiological studies that atrophy of the hippocampus is an early predictor of dementia [Apostolova et al.,, 2006; Juottonen, Laasko, Partanen and Soinen, 1999]. Therefore, persons with Stage I and Stage II do not have dementia but have some problems with metamemory and often seek advice at this early stage.

However, as the degenerative process progresses, there is severe destruction of the transentorhinal and the entorhinal regions (Stage III) with changes in the hippocampus and also to the amygdala, and then at a later stage in the temporal and insular proneocortices and neocortices (Stage IV). Indeed, it has been shown that persons with stage III and IV pathology exhibit amnestic MCI [Jicha et al., 2006; Petersen et al., 2006]. The blocking of flow to the hippocampus but continuing flow to amygdala may explain the high initial presence of anxiety, a manifest of amygdalar overactivity [Lange and Irie, 2004]. (see figure 3).

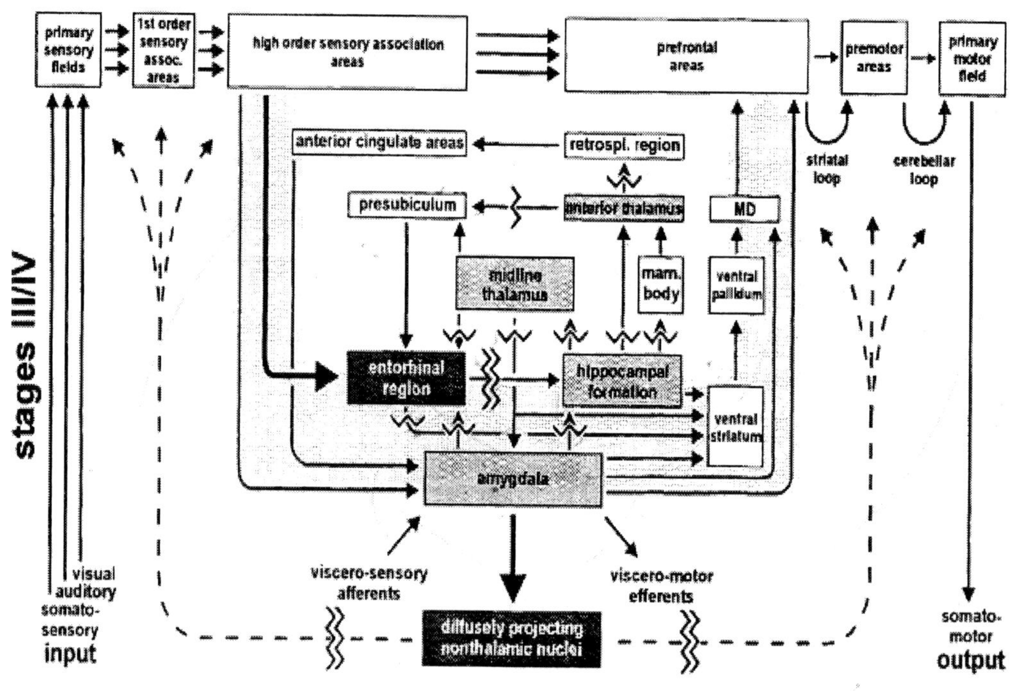

Figure 3. Model of development of interference of information transfer according to Braak and Braak Stages III/IV (Reprinted with permission from Braak, Del Tredici and Braak, 2003).

By stages V (extensive damage of the neocortex) and VI (penetration of the destruction to the primary fields), a diagnosis of dementia is made and there is an absence of amgdalar overactivity. In the author's present unpublished study [Sinoff, 2007], the prevalence of anxiety decreased over two years from 36% to 8% and depression from 13.9% to 8%, findings similar to those reported by researchers from Amsterdam who concluded that the neuropsychiatric symptoms of depression and anxiety increase in the early phase of cognitive decline and decrease as cognitive function declines [Bierman et al., 2007].

Results from the Mayo Clinic of Petersen's group showed that volume changes in the hippocampus, entorhinal cortex, whole brain and ventricule were all predictive of conversion from normal to MCI and from MCI to dementia [Jack et al., 2004] and recently these changes were reported to occur up to 4 years prior to the diagnosis of MCI [Smith et al., 2007]. This tends to support the neuropathological findings of Braak that the initial pathology is occurring in the entorhinal cortex [Albert, 2003]. Recently Devanand and co-researchers [2007] reported comparable findings in their study of MCI subjects supporting the concept that the entorhinal cortex atrophies before the hippocampus in incipient AD.

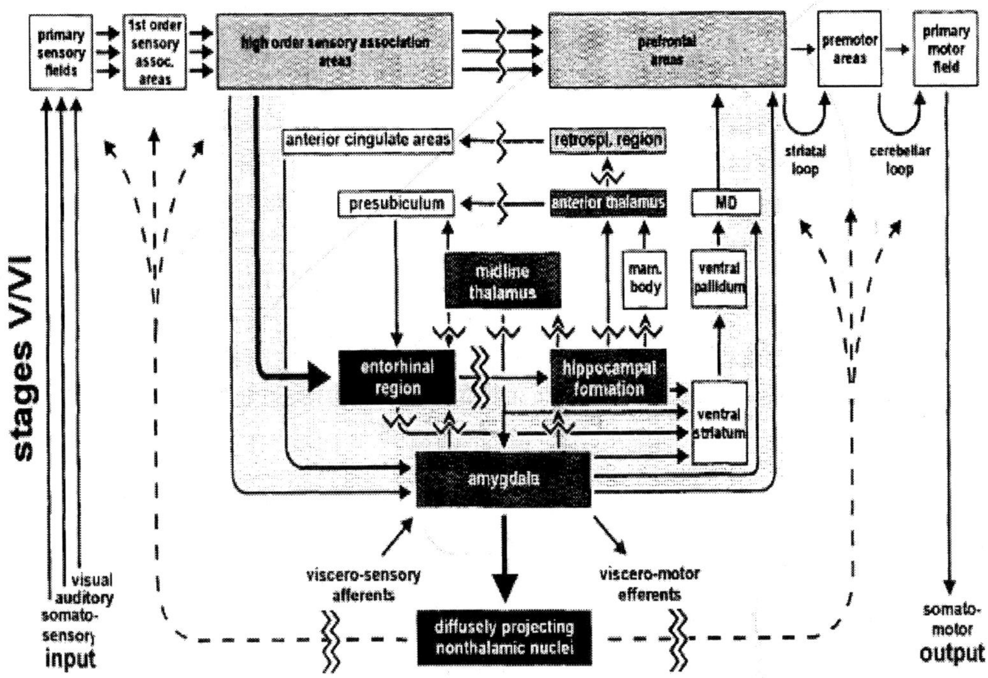

Figure 4. Model of development of interference of information transfer according to Braak and Braak Stages V/VI (Reprinted with permission from Braak, Del Tredici and Braak, 2003).

Few studies have examined amygdalar volume changes. According to Braak, Del Tredici and Braak [2003], initially the amygdala is not affected by the degenerative process (see above illustration), but at later stages, it too undergoes degeneration. In a study by Den Heijer and colleagues [2006], it was found that both hippocampal and amygdalar volumes were strongly associated with the risk of dementia over an extended period of time.

Studies investigating the changes in hippocampal volume in depression show conflicting findings. Hickie and co-workers [2005] reported reduction of hippocampal volume in persons suffering from depression and memory loss, but Hastings and colleagues found no difference in the hippocampal volume in depressed patients (with no memory loss) and normal controls [Hastings, Parsey, Oquendo, Arango and Mann, 2004]. On the other hand, researchers from the University of Gottingen, Germany found that those with depression had significantly enlarged amygdala size and reduced hippocampal size [Lange and Irie, 2004; Weniger, Lange and Irie, 2006] as did Diamond and colleagues [2004] who reported hippocampal processing is impaired and amygdaloid processing enhanced in both mood disorders, depression and anxiety, thus reinforcing the concept that depression-preceding dementia is actually secondary to the process of memory impairment and a clinical manifestation of awareness of the subject's metamemory problems. Wilson and colleagues [2007] from Rush Alzheimer's Disease Center found that neuroticism was associated with loss of cognition and concluded that psychological distress might be an early sign of the pathology of Alzheimer disease.

CONCLUSION

In conclusion, it can be hypothesized that at the very early stages of subjective memory loss, a person is aware of his memory problem and becomes anxious related to the degenerative process. The flow of information along the entorhinal cortex to the hippocampus is interrupted, nevertheless the hippocampus is still receiving information by means of the alternative pathway via the amygdala, causing amygdala hyperactivity. This may explain the findings of this author's initial study [Sinoff and Werner, 2003] where it was found that those turning for a geriatric assessment in the community with memory problems had high incidence of anxiety and were probably at Braak Stages I or II with mild distortion of information flow to the hippocampus, which is the primary area of the brain related to memory. The flow of information may be increased via the alternative pathway via the amygdala, the area related to mood disturbances. In this author's present unpublished study [Sinoff, 2007] those with a diagnosis of MCI, Braak Stage III or maybe stage IV, still have a high prevalence of anxiety at initial onset but during the study period, the rate of anxiety decreases as the subjects became demented.

However, the presence of anxiety in itself was not a predictor of future cognitive decline even though there was a trend as shown below in the Kaplan-Meyer analysis [Sinoff, 2007] (see . It may require an extended study period to discover if those with MCI accompanied by anxiety develop greater rate of cognitive decline after many years.

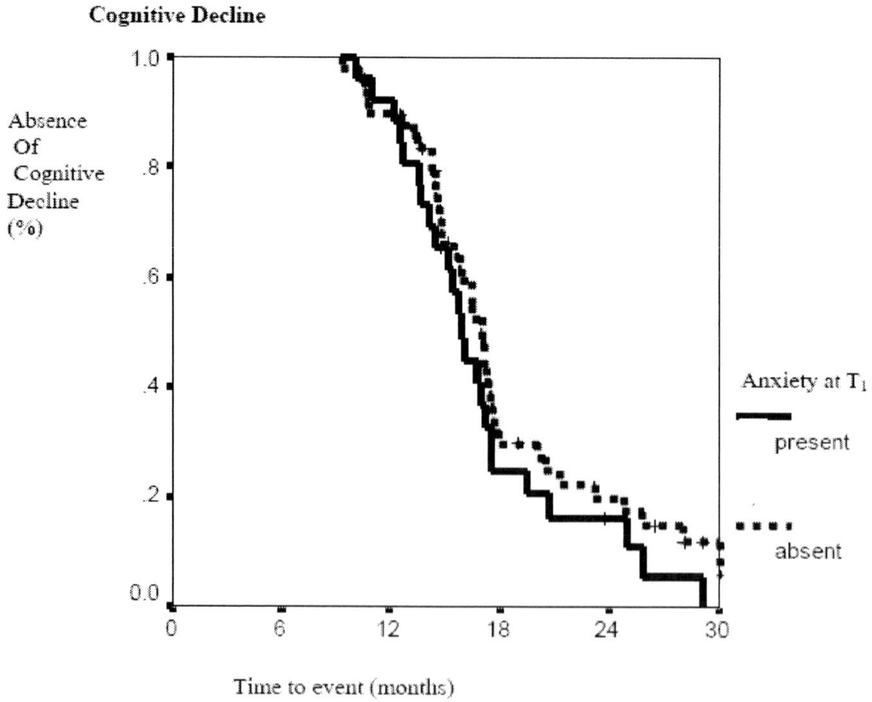

Chi-square= .466

Kaplan-Meier Survival Analysis with Cognitive Decline as end-point by presence or absence of anxiety (Sinoff, 2007).

Since MCI is defined as a transitional state between normal aging and dementia, with a conversion rate of about 20-30% per annum, a clinician should have the means at his disposal to predict the converters, since the earlier one starts therapy, the more effective the treatment is in delaying the onset of dementia. Yet, we are studying an ill-defined clinical entity with no clear gold-standard for diagnosis [Ganguli, 2006]. In truth, it is probable that the dementing process may be detected even before the MCI stage [Storandt et al., 2006], a fact emphasizing the need for finding the early predictors of cognitive decline. Many approaches have been and are being investigated including neuroimaging, biomarkers, genetics and clinical neuropsychological testing. The neuropsychiatric states, depression and anxiety, have also been examined as predictors. Depression has been reported to be a clinical predictor for future cognitive decline in persons with MCI [Crowe et al., 2006] and recently also anxiety was found to be a predictor in subjects in a community study [Palmer et al., 2007; Sinoff and Werner, 2003]. However, anxiety was unproven to be a predictor of future cognitive decline in the two year follow-up of MCI patients [Sinoff, 2007]. These differences may be explained by the blurred boundaries existing between MCI and normal aging at one end and MCI and dementia at the other [Petersen and Morris, 2003].

Theoretically, early MCI is a prodromal stage where the person is aware of his memory loss but minimal clinical evidence is present. By means of the neuroanatomical model explained above [Braak, Del Tredici and Braak, 2003], at this early stage of MCI where disturbances of flow of information to the hippocampus via the entorhinal cortex exist, anxiety may be the presenting feature related to the over-stimulation of the amygdala via the alternative pathway. Since, the degenerative process continues in the brain, it is to be expected that future cognitive decline would be present on follow-up. So anxiety at this early stage is the initial clinical manifestation of the dementing process [Cummings, 2003]. At the later stage of MCI, anxiety is present but the overlap of MCI is now with dementia, and most of the subjects may already be in the stage of early dementia. They manifest rather with cognitive decline and the anxiety is an accompaniment to the process. This explains the inability of anxiety, which is a result of the dementia, to predict further cognitive decline since all persons with late MCI stage have a greater tendency for cognitive decline. Though in effect there does seem to be a trend that persons with MCI and anxiety do have a greater risk of further cognitive decline.

REFERENCES

Aalten, P., de Vugt, M.E., Jaspers, N., Jolles, J. and Verhey, F.R. (2005). The course of neuropsychiatric symptoms in dementia: Part II: relationships among behavioral sub-syndromes and the influence of clinical variables. *International Journal of Geriatric Psychiatry, 20*, 531-536.

Adak, S., Illouz, K., Gorma, W., Tandon, R., Zimmerman, E.A., Guariglia, R., Moore, M.M. and Kaye, J.A. (2004). Predicting the rate of cognitive decline in aging and early Alzheimer disease. *Neurology, 63*, 108-114.

Albert, M.S. (2003). Detection of very early Alzheimer disease through neuroimaging. *Alzheimer Disease and Associated Disorders, 17 (Supplement 2),* S63-S65.

Alexopoulos, P., Grimmer, T., Perneczky, R., Domes, G. and Kurz, A. (2006). Progression to dementia in clinical subtypes of mild cognitive impairment. *Dementia and Geriatric Cognitive Disorders, 22,* 27-34.

American Psychiatric Association.(1994). *Diagnostic and Statistical Manual of Mental Disorders, Fourth Edition.* Washington, D.C.: American Psychiatric Association.

Amieva, H., Letenneur, L., Dartigues, J-F., Rouch-Leroyer, I., Sourgen, C., D'Alchée-Biré, F., Dib, M., Barberger-Gateau, P. and Orgogozoz, J-M. Fabriguole, C. (2004). Annual rate and predictors of conversion of conversion to dementia in subjects presenting mild cognitive impairment criteria defined according to a population-based study. *Dementia and Geriatric Cognitive Disorders, 18,* 87-93.

Apostolova, L.G., Dutton, R.A., Dinov, R.A., Dinov, I.D., Hayashi, K.M., Toga, A.W., Cummings, J.L. and Thompson, P.M. (2006). Conversion of mild cognitive impairment to Alzheimer disease predicted by hippocampal atrophy maps. *Archives of Neurology, 63,* 693-699.

Berger, A-K., Fratiglioni, L., Forsell, Y., Winblad, B. and Bäckman., L. (1999). The occurrence of depressive symptoms in the preclinical phase of AD. A population-based study. *Neurology, 53,* 1998–2002.

Bierman, E.J.M., Comijs, H.C., Jonker, C. and Beekman, A.T.F. (2005). Effects of anxiety versus depression on cognition in later life. *American Journal of Geriatric Psychiatry, 13,* 686-693.

Bookheimer, S.Y., Strojwas, M.H., Cohen, M.S., Saunders, A.M., Pericak-Vance, M.A., Mazziotta, J.C. and Small, G.W. (2000). Patterns of brain activation in people at risk for Alzheimer's disease. *New England Journal of Medicine, 343*, 450-456.

Boyle, P.A., Wilson, R.S., Aggarwal, N.T., Tang, Y. and Bennett, D.A. (2006). Mild Cognitive Impairment. Risk of Alzheimer disease and rate of cognitive decline. *Neurology, 67,* 441-445.

Braak, H., Del Tredici, K. and Braak, E. (2003). Spectrum of Pathology. In R.C. Petersen (Editor): *Mild Cognitive Impairment. Aging to Alzheimer's Disease.* Oxford University Press: New York. Chapter 8, pages 149-204.

Busse, A., Bischkopf, J., Riedel-Heller, S.G. and Angermeyer, M.C. (2003). Subclassification for mild cognitive impairment: prevalence and predictive validity. *Psychological Medicine, 33,* 1029-1038.

Chertkow, H. (2002). Mild cognitive impairment. *Current Opinion in Neurology, 15,* 401-407.

Christensen, H., Henderson, A.S., Korten, A.E., Jorm, A.F., Jacomb, P.A. and Mackinnon, A.J. (1997). ICD-10 mild cognitive disorder: Its outcome three years later. *International Journal of Geriatric Psychiatry, 12,* 581–586.

Clare, L., Wilson, B.A., Carter, G., Breen, K., Bernos, G.E. and Hodges, J.R. (2002). Depression and anxiety in memory clinic attenders and their carers: Implications for evaluating the effectiveness of cognitive rehabilitation interventions. *International Journal of Geriatric Psychiatry, 17,* 962-967.

Collie, A. and Maruff, P. (2000). The neuropsychology of preclinical Alzheimer's disease and mild cognitive impairment. *Neuroscience and Biobehavioural Reviews, 24,* 365–374.

Crowe, M., Andel, R., Wadley, V., Cook, S., Unverzagt, F., Marsiske, M. and Ball, K. (2006). Subjective cognitive function and decline among older adults. *International Journal of Geriatric Psychiatry, 21,* 1187-1192.

Cummings, J.L. (2003). Neuropsychiatric Symptoms. In: R.C. Petersen (Editor). *Mild Cognitive Impairment. Aging to Alzheimer's Disease.* Oxford University Press: New York. Chapter 3, pages 41-61.

Cutler, S.J. and Hodgson, L.G. (1996). Anticipatory dementia: A link between memory appraisals and concerns about developing Alzheimer's disease. *The Gerontologist, 36 (5),* 657–664

DeCarli, C., Frisoni, G.B., Clark, C.M., Harvey, D., Grundman, M., Petersen, R.C., Thal, L.J., Jin, S., Jack Jr., C.R., Scheltens, P. for the Alzheimer's Disease Cooperative Study Group. (2007). Qualitative estimates of medial temporal atrophy as a predictor of progression from mild cognitive impairment to dementia. *Archives of Neurology, 64,* 108-115.

DeKosky, S. (2003). Early intervention is the key to successful management of Alzheimer disease. *Alzheimer Disease and Associated Disorders, 17 (Supplement 4),* S99-S104.

DeKosky, S.T. and Marek, K. (2003). Looking backward to move forward: Early detection of neurodegenerative disorders. *Science, 302,* 830-834.

de Leon, M.J., DeSanti, S., Zinkowski, R., Mehta, P.D., Pratico, D., Segal, S., Rusinek, H., Li, J., Tsui, W., Saint Louis, L.A., Clark, C.M., Tarshish, C., Li, Y., Lair, L., Javier, E., Rich, K., Lesbre, P., Mosconi, L., Reisberg, B., Sadowski, M., DeBernadis, J.F., Kerkman, D.J., Hampel, H., Wahlund, L.O. and Davies, P. (2006). Longitudinal CSF and MRI biomarkers improve the diagnosis of mid cognitive impairment. *Neurobiology of Aging, 27,* 394-401.

DeLuca, A.K., Lenze, E.J., Mulsant, B.H., Butters, M.A., Karp, J.F., Dew, M.A., Pollock, B.g., Shear, K., Houck, P.R. and Reynolds III, C.F. (2005). Comorbid anxiety disorder in late life depression: association with memory decline over four years. *International Journal of Geriatric Psychiatry, 20,* 848-854.

Den Heijer, T., Geerlings, M.I., Hoebeek, F.E., Hofman, A., Koudstaal, P.J. and Breteler, M.M. (2006). Use of hippocampal and amygdalar volumes on magnetic resonance imaging to predict dementia in cognitively intact elderly people. *Archives of General Psychiatry, 63,* 57-62.

Derouesné, C., Thibault, S., Lagha-Pierucci, S., Baudouin-Madec, V., Ancri, D. and Lacomblez, L. (1999). Decreased awareness of cognitive deficits in patients with mild dementia of the Alzheimer type. *International Journal of Geriatric Psychiatry, 14,* 1019–1030.

Devanand, D.P., Pradhaban, G., Liu, X., Khandji, A., De Santi, S., Segal. S., Rusinek, H., Pelton, G.H., Honig, L.S., Mayeux, R., Stern, Y., Tabert, M.H. and de Leon, M.J. (2007). Hippocampal and entorhinal atrophy in mild cognitive impairment. *Neurology, 68,* 828-836.

Devanand, D.P., Sano, M., Tang M-X, Taylor, S., Gurland, B.J., Wilder, D., Stern, Y. and Mayeux, R. (1996). Depressed mood and the incidence of Alzheimer's disease in the elderly living in the community. *Archives of General Psychiatry, 53,* 175–182.

Diamond, D.M., Campbell, A., Park, C.R. and Vouimba, R.M. (2004). Preclinical research on stress, memory, and the brain in the development of pharmacotherapy for depression. *European Neuropsychopharmacology, 14 (Supplement 5),* S491-S496.

Di Carlo, A., Baldereschi M., Amaducci, L., Lepore, V., Bracco, L., Maggi, S., bonaiuto, S., Perssinotto, E., Scarlato, G., Farchi,G., and Inzitari, D. for the Italian Longitudinal Study on Aging Working Group. (2002). Incidence of dementia, Alzheimer's disease and vascular dementia in Italy. The LSA study. *Journal of the American Geriatrics Society, 50,* 41-48.

Dierckx, E., Engelborghs, S., De Raedt, R., De Deyn, P.P. and Ponjaert-Kristoffersen, I. (2007). Mild cognitive impairment: what's in a name? *Gerontology, 53(1),* 28-35.

Edwards, E.R., Lindquist, K. and Yaffe, K. (2004). Clinical profile and course of cognitively normal patients evaluated in memory disorders clinics. *Neurology, 62,* 1639-1642.

Feldman, H., Scheltens, P., Scarpini, E., Hermann, N., Mesenbrink, P., Mancione, L., Tekin, S., Lane, R. and Ferris, S. (2004). Behavioral symptoms in mild cognitive impairment. *Neurology, 62,* 1199-1201.

Flicker, C., Ferris, S.H. and Reisberg, B. (1991). Mild cognitive impairment in the elderly: Predictors of dementia. *Neurology, 41,* 1006-1009.

Forsell, Y., Palmer, K. and Fratiglioni, L. (2003). Psychiatric symptoms/ syndromes in elderly persons with mild cognitive impairment. Data from a cross-sectional study. *Acta Neurologica Scandanavica, 107 (Supplement 179),* 25-28.

Friedrich, M.J. (1999). Mild cognitive impairment raises Alzheimer disease risk. *Journal of the American Medical Association, 282 (7),* 621–622.

Gabryelewicz, T., Styczynska, M., Luczywek, E., Barczak, A., Pfeffer, A., Androsiuk, W., Chodakowska-Zebrowska, M., Wasiak, B., Peplonska, B. and Basrcikowska, M. (2007). The rate of conversion of mild cognitive impairment to dementia: predictive role of depression. *International Journal of Geriatric Psychiatry, 22(6),* 563-567.

Galasko, D. (2001). New approaches to diagnose and treat Alzheimer's disease. *Clinics in Geriatric Medicine, 17 (2),* 393-410.

Ganguli, M. (2006). Mild cognitive impairment and the 7 uses of epidemiology. *Alzheimer Disease and Associated Disorders, 20 (Supplement 2),* S52-S57.

Geda, Y.E., Knopman, D.S., Mrazek, D.A., Jicha, G.A., Smith, G.E., Negash, S., Boeve, B.F., Ivnik, R.J., Petersen, R.C., Pankratz, V.S. and Rocca, W.A. (2006). Depression, apolipoprotein E genotype, and the incidence of mild cognitive impairment: a prospective cohort study. *Archives of Neurology, 63 (3),* 435 – 440.

Graham, J.E., Rockwood, K., Beattie, L., Eastwood, R., Gauthier, S., Tuokko, H. and McDowell, I. (1997). Prevalence and severity of cognitive impairment with and without dementia in an elderly population. *Lancet, 349,* 1793-1796.

Green, R.C., Cupples, L.A., Kurz, A., Auerbach, S., Go, R., Sadovnick, D., Duara, R., Kukull, W.A., Chui, H., Edeki, T., Griffith, P.A., Friedland, R.P., Bachman, D. and Farrer, L. (2003). Depression as a risk factor for Alzheimer's disease. The Mirage Study. *Archives of Neurology, 60,* 753-759.

Griffith, H.R., Netson, K.L., Harrell, L.E., Zamrini, E.Y., Brockington, J.C. and Marson, D.C. (2006). Amnestic mild cognitive impairment: Diagnostic outcomes and clinical prediction over a two-year period. *Journal of the International Neuropsychological Society, 12,* 166-175.

Grundman, M., Petersen, R.C., Ferris, S.H., Thomas, R.G., Aisen, P.S., Bennett, D.A., Foster, N.L., Jack, C.R., Galasko, D.G., Doody, R., Kaye, J., Sano, M., Mohs, R., Gauthier, S., Kim, H.T., Jin, S., Schultz, A.N., Schafer, K., Mulnard, R., Thal, L.J., for the Alzheimer Disease Cooperative Study. (2004). Mild cognitive impairment can be distinguished from Alzheimer disease and normal aging for clinical trials. *Archives of Neurology, 61,* 59-66.

Guillozet, A.L., Weintraub, S., Mash, D.C. and Mesulaem, M.M. (2003). Neurofibrillary tangles, amyloid, and memory in aging and mild cognitive impairment. *Archives of Neurology, 60,* 729 – 736.

Hänninen, T., Hallikainen, M., Toumainen, S., Vanhanen, M. and Soininen, H. (2002). Prevalence of mild cognitive impairment: a population-based study in elderly subjects. *Acta Neurologica Scandanavica, 106,* 148-154.

Harwood, D.G., Barker, W.W., Ownby, R.L., and Duara, R. (2000). Relationship of behavioral and psychological symptoms to cognitive impairment and functional status in Alzheimer's disease. *International Journal of Geriatric Psychiatry, 15,* 393-400.

Hastings, R.S., Parsey, R.V., Oquendo, M.A., Arango, V. and Mann, J.J. (2004). Volumetric analysis of the prefrontal cortex, amygdala, and hippocampus in major depression. *Neuropsychopharmacology, 29,* 952-959.

Herukka, S.K., Hallikainen, M., Soininen, H. and Pirttila, T. (2005). CSF Abeta42 and tau or phosphorylated tau and prediction of progressive mild cognitive impairment. *Neurology, 64,* 1294-1297.

Hickie, I., Naismith, S., Ward, P.B., Turner, K., Scott, E., Mitchell, P., Wilhelm, K. and Parker, G. (2005). Reduced hippocampal volumes and memory loss in patients with early- and late-onset depression. *British Journal of Psychiatry, 186,* 197-202.

Hodges, J.R., Erzinçlioğlu, S. and Patterson, K. (2006). Evolution of cognitive deficits and conversion to dementia in patients with mild cognitive impairment: A very-long-term follow-up study. *Dementia and Geriatric Cognitive Disorders, 21,* 380-391.

Huang, C., Wahlund, L-O., Dierks, T., Julin, P., Winbald, B. and Jelic, V. (2000). Discrimination of Alzheimer's disease and mild cognitive impairment by equivalent EEG sources; A cross-sectional and longitudinal study. *Clinical Neurophysiology, 111,* 1961-1967.

Hwang, T.J., Masterman, D.L., Ortiz, F., Fairbanks, L.A. and Cummings, J.L. (2004). Mild cognitive impairment is associated with characteristic neuropsychiatric symptoms. *Alzheimer Disease and Associated Disorders, 18,* 17-21.

Jack Jr., C.R., Shiung, M.M., Gunter, J.L., O'Brien, P.C., Weigand, S.D., Knopman, D.S., Boeve, B.F., Smith, G.E., Cha, R.H., Tangalos, E.G. and Petersen, R.C. (2004). Comparison of different MRI brain atrophy rate measures with clinical disease progression in AD. *Neurology, 62*, 591-600.

Jicha, G.A., Parisi, J.E., Dickson, D.W., Johnson, K., Cha ,R., Ivnik, R.J., Tangalos, E.G., Boeve, B.F., Knopman, D.S., Braak, H. and Petersen, R.C. (2006). Neuropathological outcome of mild cognitive impairment following progression to clinical dementia. *Archives of Neurology,* 63, 674-681.

Jorm, A.F., Christensen, H., Korten, A.E., Henderson, A.S., Jacomb, P.A. and Mackinnon, A. (1997). Do cognitive complaints either predict future cognitive decline or reflect past cognitive decline? A longitudinal study of an elderly community sample. *Psychological Medicine, 27,* 91–98.

Juottonen, K., Laakso, P., Partanen, K. and Soininen, H. (1999). Compartive MR analysis of the etorhinal cortex and hippocampus in diagnosing Alzheimer disease. *American Journal of Neuroradiology, 20,* 139-144.

Karlawish, J.H.T., Casarett, D.J., James, B.D., Tenhave, T., Clark, C.M. and Asch, D.A. (2003). Why would caregivers not want to treat their relative's Alzheimer's disease? *Journal of the American Geriatrics Society, 51*, 1391-1397.

Lange, C. and Irle, E. (2004). Enlarged amygdala volume and reduced hippocampal volume in young women with major depression. *Psychological Medicine, 34,* 1059- 1064.

Larrieu, S., Letenneur, L., Orgogozo, J.M., Fabrigoule, C., Amieva, H., Le Carret, N., Barberger-Gateau, P. and Dartigues, D.F. (2002). Incidence and outcome of mild cognitive impairment in a population-based prospective cohort. *Neurology, 59,* 1594-1599.

Lanctôt, K.L., Herrmann, N., Yau, K.K., Khan, L.R., Liu, B.A., LouLou, M.M. and Einarson, T.R. (2003). Efficacy and safety of cholinesterase inhibitors in Alzheimer's disease: a meta-analysis. *Canadian Medical Association Journal, 169,* 557-564.

Lee, J.S., Potter, G.G., Wagner, H.R., Welsh-Bohmer, K.A. and Steffens, D.C. (2007). Persistent mild cognitive impairment in geriatric depression. *International Psychogeriatrics, 19 (1),* 125-135.

Li, Y.-S., Meyer, J.S. and Thornby, J. (2001). Longitudinal follow-up of depressive symptoms among normal versus cognitively impaired elderly. *International Journal of Geriatric Psychiatry, 16,* 718-727.

Lyketsos, C.G., Chen, L.-S. and Anthony, J.C. (1999). Cognitive decline in adulthood: An 11.5-year follow-up of the Baltimore epidemiologic catchment area study. *American Journal of Psychiatry, 156,* 58-65.

Manly, J.J., Bell-McGinty, S., Tang, M-X., Schupf, N., Stern, Y. and Mayeux, R. (2005). Implementing diagnostic criteria and estimating frequency of mild cognitive impairment in an urban community. *Archives of Neurology, 62,* 1739-1746.

Mega, M.S., Cummings, J.L., Fiorello, T. and Gornbein, J. (1996). The spectrum of behavioral changes in Alzheimer's disease. *Neurology, 46(1),* 130-135.

Modrego, P.J., Fayed, N. and Pina, MA. (2005). Conversion from mild cognitive impairment to probable Alzheimer's disease predicted by brain magnetic resonance spectroscopy. *American Journal of Psychiatry, 162,* 667-675.

Modrego, P.J. and Ferrandez, J. (2004). Depression in patients with mild cognitive impairment increases the risk of developing dementia of Alzheimer type. A Prospective Cohort Study. *Archives of Neurology, 61,* 1290-1293.

Morris, J.C., Storandt, M., Miller, J.P., Price, J.L., Rubin, E.H. and Berg, L. (2001). Mild cognitive impairment represents early-stage Alzheimer disease. *Archives of Neurology, 58 (3),* 397-405.

Ownby, R.L., Harwood, D.G., Barker, W.W. and Duara, R. (2000). Predictors of anxiety in patients with Alzheimer disease. *Depression and Anxiety, 11,* 38-42.

Palmer, K., Berger, A.K., Monastero, R., Winblad, B., Bäckman, L. and Fratiglioni, L. (2007). Predictors of progression from mild cognitive impairment to Alzheimer disease. *Neurology, 68,* 1596-1602.

Palmer, K., Bäckman, L., Winblad, B. and Fratiglioni, L. (2003). Detection of Alzheimer's disease and dementia in the preclinical phase: population based cohort study. *British Medical Journal, 326,* 245-249.

Palmer, K., Berger, A.K., Monastero, R., Winblad, B., Bäckman, L. and Fratiglioni, L. (2007). Predictors of progression from mild cognitive impairment to Alzheimer disease. *Neurology, 68,* 1596-1602.

Pannu, J.K. and Kaszniak, A.W. (2005). Metamemory experiments in neurological populations: A review. *Neuropsychological Review, 15 (3),* 105-130.

Paterniti, S., Dufouil C, Bisserbe, J.C. and Alpérovitch, A. (1999). Anxiety, depression, psychotropic drug use and cognitive impairment. *Psychological Medicine, 29*, 421-428.

Petersen, R.C., Doody, R., Kurz, A., Mohs, R.C., Morris, J.C., Rabins, P.V., Ritchie, K., Rossor, M., Thai, L. and Winblad, B. (2001). Current concepts in mild cognitive impairment. *Archives of Neurology, 58,* 1985 – 1992.

Petersen, R.C. and Morris, J.C. (2005). Mild cognitive impairment as a clinical entity and treatment target. *Archives of Neurology, 62,* 1160-1163.

Petersen, R.C. and Morris, J.C. (2003). Clinical Features. In: R.C. Petersen (Editor): *Mild Cognitive Impairment. Aging to Alzheimer's Disease.* Oxford University Press: New York. Chapter 2, pages 15-39.

Petersen, R.C., Parisi, J.E., Dickson, D.W., Johnson, K.A., Knopman, D.S., Boeve, B.F., Jicha, G.A., Ivnik, R.J., Smith, G.E., Tanglos, E.G., Braak, H. and Kokmen, E. (2006). Neuropathological features of amnestic mild cognitive impairment. *Archives of Neurology, 63,* 665-672.

Petersen, R.C., Smith, G.E., Ivnik, R.J., Kokmen, E. and Tangalos, E.G. (1994). Memory function in very early Alzheimer's disease. *Neurology, 44,* 867-872.

Petersen, R.C., Smith, G.E., Waring, S.C., Ivnik, R.J., Tangalos, E.G. and Kokmen, E. (1999). Mild cognitive impairment: Clinical characterization and outcome. *Archives of Neurology, 56(3),* 303-308.

Petersen, R.C., Stevens, J.C., Ganguli, M., Tangalos, E.G., Cummings, J.E. and DeKosky, S.T. (2001). Early detection of dementia: Mild cognitive impairment (an evidence-based review). *Neurology, 56,* 1133-1142.

Ponds, R.W.H.M. and Jolles, J. (1996). Memory complaints in elderly people: The role of memory abilities, metamemory, depression, and personality. *Educational Gerontology, 22,* 341-357.

Rasquin, S.M.C., Lodder, J., Visser, P.J., Lousberg, R. and Verhey, F.R.J. (2005). Predictive accuracy of MCI subtypes for Alzheimer's disease and vascular dementia in subjects with mild cognitive impairment: a 2-year follow-up study. *Dementia and Geriatric Cognitive Disorders*, *19*, 113-119.

Ritchie, K. and Touchon, J. (2000). Mild cognitive impairment: Conceptual basis and current nosological status. *The Lancet, 355*, 225–228.

Rubin, E.H., Veiel, L.L., Kinscherf, D.A., Morris, J.C. and Storandt, M. (2001). Clinically significant depressive symptoms and very mild to mild dementia of the Alzheimer type. *International Journal of Geriatric Psychiatry, 16,* 694-701.

Ryu, S-H., Katona, C., Rive, B. and Livingston, G. (2005). Persistence of and changes in neuropsychiatric symptoms in Alzheimer's disease over 6 months. The LASER-AD study. *American Journal of Geriatric Psychiatry, 13,* 976-983.

Sadik, K. and Wilcock, G. (2003). The increasing burden of Alzheimer disease. *Alzheimer Disease and Associated Disorders, 17 (Supplement 3),* S75-S79.

Schneider, L.S. (1996). Overview of generalized anxiety disorder in the elderly. *Journal of Clinical Psychiatry, 57 (Supplement 7),* 34–45.

Shah, Y., Tangalos, E.G. and Petersen, R.C. (2000). Mild cognitive impairment. When is it a precursor to Alzheimer's disease. *Geriatrics, 55 (9),* 62–68.

Sinoff, G. (2007). Anxiety in persons with Mild Cognitive Impairment: Is it a predictor of future cognitive decline? *Thesis (Ph.D. - University of Haifa, The Graduate Students Authority, The Committee for Doctoral, 2007)*. Universitat Hefah – Dissertations (Ph.D.). ULI (The Israel Union Catalog) Number: 00812093.

Sinoff, G. and Werner, P. (2003). Anxiety disorder and accompanying subjective memory loss in the elderly as a predictor of future cognitive decline. *International Journal of Geriatric Psychiatry, 18,* 951-959.

Small, G.W, Chen, S.T., Komo, S., Ercoli, L., Miller, K., Siddarth, P., Kaplan, A., Doisey, D., Lavretsky, H., Saxena, S. and Bookheimer, S.Y. (2001). Memory self-appraisal and depressive symptoms in people at genetic risk for Alzheimer's disease. *International Journal of Geriatric Psychiatry, 16,* 1071-1077.

Smith, C.D., Chebrolu, H., Wekstein, D.R., Schmitt, F.A., Jicha, G.A., Cooper, G. and Markerbery, W.R. (2007). Brain structural alterations before mild cognitive impairment. *Neurology, 68,* 1268-1273.

Solfrizzi, V., DelIntrono, A., Colacicco, A.M., Capurso, C., Del Parigi, S., Caselli, R.J., Scapicchio, P.L., Scafato, E., Gandin, C., Capurso, A., Panza, F., for the Italian Longitudinal Study on Aging Working Group. (2007). Incident occurrence of depressive symptoms among patients with mild cognitive impairment – the Italian Longitudinal Study of Aging. *Dementia and Geriatric Cognitive Disorders,* 55-64.

Starkstein, S.E., Jorge, R., Petracca, G. and Robinson, R.G. (2007). The construct of generalized anxiety disorder in Alzheimer disease. *American Journal of Geriatric Psychiatry, 15,* 42-49.

Storandt, M., Grant, E.A., Miller, J.P. and Morris, J.C. (2006). Longitudinal course and neuropathologic outcomes in original vs revised MCI and in pre-MCI. *Neurology, 67,* 467-478.

Stoub, T.R., de Toledo-Morrell, L., Stebbins, G.T., Leurgans, S., Bennett, D.A. and Shah, R.C. (2006). Hippocampal disconnection contributes to memory dysfunction in individuals at risk for Alzheimer's disease. *Proceedings of the National Academy of Sciences, 103,* 10041-10045.

Tatsch, M.F., de Campos Bottino, C.M., Azevedo, D., Hototian, S.R., Moscoso, M.A., Folquitto, J.C., Scalco, A.Z. and Louzã, M.R. (2006). Neuropsychiatric symptoms in Alzheimer disease and cognitively impaired nondemented elderly from a community based sample in Brazil: Prevalence and relationship with dementia severity. *American Journal of Geriatric Psychiatry, 14,* 438-445.

Tian, J., Bucks, R.S., Haworth, J. and Wilcock, G. (2003). Neuropsychological prediction of conversion to dementia from questionable dementia: statistically significant but not yet clinically useful. *Journal of Neurology, Neurosurgery and Psychiatry, 74*, 433-438.

Tschanz, J.T., Welsh-Bohmer, K.A., Lyketsos, C.G., Corcoran, C., Green, R.C., Hayden, K., Norton, M.C., Zandi, P.P., Toone, L., West, N.A., Breitner, J.C. and the Cache County Investigators. (2006). Conversion to dementia from mild cognitive disorder. The Cache County Study. *Neurology, 67*, 229-234.

Tuokko, H., Frerichs, R., Graham, J., Rockwood. K., Kristjansson, B., Fisk, J., Bergman, H., Kozma, A. and McDowell, I. (2003). Five-year follow-up of cognitive impairment with no dementia. *Archives of Neurology, 60,* 577-582.

Visser, P.J., Kester, A., Jolles, J. and Verhey, F. (2006). Ten-year risk of dementia in subjects with mild cognitive impairment. *Neurology, 67,* 1201-1207.

Visser, P.J., Verhey, F.R.J., Ponds, R.W.H.M., Cruts, M., van Broeckhoven, C.L. and Jolles, J. (2000). Course of objective memory impairment in non-demented subjects attending a memory clinic and predictors of outcome. *International Journal of Geriatric Psychiatry, 15,* 363-372.

Visser, P.J., Verhey, F.R.J., Ponds, R.W.H.M., Kester, A. and Jolles, J. (2000). Distinction between preclinical Alzheimer's disease and depression. *Journal of the American Geriatrics Society, 48,* 479–484.

Wahlund, L-O., Pihlstrand, E. and Jönhagen, M.E. (2003). Mild cognitive impairment: Experience from a memory clinic. *Acta Neurologica Scandanavica, 107 (Supplement 179)*, 21-24.

Waite, L.M., Broe, G.A., Grayson, D.A. and Creasey, H. (2001). Preclinical syndromes predict dementia: the Sydney older persons study. *Journal of Neurology, Neurosurgery and Psychiatry, 71*, 296-302.

Weniger, G., Lange, C. and Irle, E. (2006). Abnormal size of the amygdala predicts impaired emotional memory in major depressive disorder. *Journal of Affective Disorders, 94*, 219-229.

Wilson, R.S., Arnold, S.E., Schneider, J.A., Li, Y. and Bennett, D.A. (2007). Chronic distress, age-related neuropathology, and late-life dementia. *Psychosomatic Medicine, 69*, 47-53.

Wilson, R.S., Barnes, L.L., Mendes de Leon, C.F., Aggarwal, N.T., Schneider, J.S., Bach, J., Pilat, J., Beckett, L.A., Arnold, S.E., Evans, D.A. and Bennett, D.A. (2002). Depressive symptoms, cognitive decline, and risk of AD in older persons. *Neurology, 59,* 364-370.

Winblad, B., Palmer, K., Kivipelto, M., Jelic, V., Fratiglioni, L., Wahlund, L.O., Nordberg, A., Bäckman, L., Albert, M., Almkvist, O., Arai, H., Basun, H., Blennow, K., de Leon, M., DeCarli, C., Erkinjuntti, T., Giacobini, E., Graff, C., Hardy, J., Jack, C., Jorm, A., Ritchie, K., van Duijn, C., Visser, P. and Petersen, R.C. (2004). Mild cognitive impairment – beyond controversies, towards a consensus: report of the International Working Group on Mild Cognitive Impairment. *Journal of Internal Medicine, 256,* 240-246.

Wolf, H., Jelic, V., Gertz, H-J., Nordberg, A., Julin, P. and Wahlund, L-O. (2003). A critical discussion of the role of neuroimaging in mild cognitive impairment. *Acta Neurologica Scandanavica, 107 (Supplement 179),* 52-76.

Zanetti, M., Ballabio, C., Abbate, C., Cutaia, C., Vergani, C. and Bergamschini, L. (2006). Mild cognitive impairment subtypes and vascular dementia in community-dwelling elderly people: A 3-year follow-up study. *Journal of the American Geriatrics Society, 54,* 580-586.

Zaudig, M. (2002). Mild cognitive impairment in the elderly. *Current Opinion in Psychiatry, 15,* 387-398.

In: Psychiatric Research Trends: Dreams and Geriatric Psychiatry ISBN 978-1-60741-760-6
Editors: Daniella M. Montez, pp.101-115

Chapter 6

NEUROBIOLOGY OF UNCONSCIOUS PROCESSES DURING WAKING AND DREAMING

Claude Gottesmann[1]
Département de Biologie, Faculté des Sciences,
Université de Nice-Sophia Antipolis, Nice, France

The conscious processes that take place during waking have been studied for many years, and research into their neurobiological basis has made great progress with the successive advances of electrophysiological, pharmacological, neurochemical and neuroimaging techniques; these advances follow thousands-of-years-old observations of psychomimetic plant utilization, and the uncertain application of psychosurgery in the forties and fifties (uncertain due to the virtual absence of previous relevant fundamental research). In contrast, the notion of unconscious mental activities, i.e., those which escape the knowledge of the subject, is more recent: while it was alluded to by Fechner (Fechner, 1848) and Helmholz (Helmholtz, 1860), it was first fully developed by Freud. Freud initially introduced the topic in a letter to Fliess, in which he developed the idea of a psychological censorship that would parallel the political censorship of the press (Freud, 1897). He subsequently published his main analysis of repressed unconscious processes that are controlled by a censorship mechanism (going beyond normal mental content that is momentarily absent from consciousness but accessible by recall (Kandel, 1999)) in his seminal book, "The interpretation of dreams" (Freud, 1900).

During waking, repressed unconscious phenomena can first be observed by the intrusion of parapraxes, as first underlined by Freud (Freud, 1901). As noted by Laplanche and Pontalis (Laplanche and Pontalis, 2006), in German the prefix 'ver' is the denominator of words indicating unconscious intrusions during waking: das Vergessen (forgetting), das Versprechen (slip of the tongue), das Verlesen (misreading), das Verschreiben (slip of the pen), das Vergreifen (bungled action), and das Verlieren (mislaying) (p 239) (Freud, 1901). For Freud, these were indices of the partial failure of a censorship process that acts to prevent the

[1] Mail address: Cl. Gottesmann, 22, parc Lubonis 06000 Nice, France.
E-mail claude.gottesmann@unice.fr.

intrusion of repressed feelings, wishes or drives into the waking consciousness. Indeed, among the different defense mechanisms available, repression from awareness is one of the most frequently used. Another is projection, the process by which the subject expels and localizes in other(s) feelings and desires he refuses for himself. Finally, there is rationalization, a common mental process that intends to render logical or morally acceptable an idea or action whose grounds are not entirely conscious.

Today, it is of interest to analyze to what extent neurobiology can account for the unconscious processes that occur during waking and sleep. The issue is not procedural unconscious processes--which concern habits and perceptual and motor skills and which are not repressed but instead remain outside of awareness--but rather repressed or "dynamic" ones (Kandel, 1999). Indeed, it could be possible to scientifically demonstrate the relevance of Freud's theory related to defense mechanisms supported by a censorship.

To function, the brain must be activated. It was long ago demonstrated that, during waking, low voltage electroencephalographic (EEG) activity (Berger, 1929, Bremer, 1935, Bremer, 1936) is related to a regular, high neuron firing rate (Evarts, 1964, Steriade, 1996), and that both of these phenomena are related to brainstem activating processes (Moruzzi and Magoun, 1949, Steriade, 1996). Central responsiveness studies, performed by evoked potential analysis (Rossi et al., 1965), have confirmed this activated state. The more recently discovered gamma rhythm (centered on 50 c/s) is also a criterion of thalamocortical activation (Bouyer et al., 1981, Ribary et al., 1991, Steriade et al., 1996). Evidence for this crucial activation of the main structures involved in mental activities has come both from studies of neurochemical transmitters (for ref. see (Gottesmann, 1999)) and from extensive neuroimaging findings (Madsen et al., 1991, Maquet et al., 1996, Braun et al., 1997, Nofzinger et al., 1997, Maquet et al., 2004). Together, these results have confirmed the activation of the entire forebrain, and particularly the cortex, during waking.

At the same time, concomitant antagonistic yet complementary inhibitory processes also have major influences at the cortical level. First identified long ago at the cortical level based on their suppression of motor activities (Bubnoff and Heidenhain, 1881), these processes were initially identified electrophysiologically based on the inhibition of cortical neuron firing (Creutzfeldt et al., 1956) and later by virtue of the long recovery cycle of cortical evoked potentials induced by radiation stimulation (Rossi et al., 1965, Allison, 1968). The neurochemical basis of this inhibition was revealed by the application of gamma aminobutyric acid (GABA) (Krnjevic et al., 1966) as well as of dopamine, noradrenaline and serotonin, which mainly inhibit cortical neurons (Krnjevic and Phillis, 1963, Reader et al., 1979); importantly, however, these monoamines also increase the signal-to-noise ratio, thus increasing neuron performance (Foote et al., 1975 , McCormick et al., 1993). The initial interpretation of these inhibitory influences, which have been extensively studied during both waking and sleep (Evarts, 1964, Demetrescu et al., 1966), was that they seemed to be the index of a process that controls cortical functioning and that decreases or disappears during sleep (Evarts, 1964).

The simultaneous functioning of both activating and inhibitory influences in the cortex can explain why some mental contents are prevented from entering consciousness during waking (with the exception of parasitic parapraxes), as their invasion of consciousness would induce anxiety and disturb daytime behavioral adaptation. Until very recently, these assertions were only supported by still valuable old electrophysiological results (Gottesmann, 1967, Gottesmann, 1970, Gottesmann, 1971). However, recent neuroimaging results have clearly confirmed that unwanted memories can be rejected from consciousness. First, the 'suppression' (from a cognitivist perspective) and 'repression' (in psychoanalytic terminology) of unwanted memories outside of awareness has been shown by 'think/no-think' task experiments (Anderson and Green, 2001). A later study by the same group was even able to show that this process involves the dorsolateral prefrontal cortex, the ventrolateral prefrontal cortex, the anterior cingulate cortex, the dorsal premotor cortex, and the intraparietal sulcus, all of which are activated during the rejected tasks. In contrast, the activation of the hippocampus, which is involved in memory processes, is strongly decreased (Anderson et al., 2004). Still more recently, it was shown that the suppression-repression phenomenon is more efficient with negative than with non-emotional information (Depue et al., 2006). This group was also able to identify the specific brain structures involved, particularly two pathways that play a role in the erasure of memories: "The first pathway involves cognitive control by right inferior frontal gyrus (rlFG) over sensory components of memory representation, as evidenced by reduced activity in fusiform gyrus and pulvinar… A second pathway involves cognitive control by right middle frontal gyrus (rMFG) over memory processes and emotional components of memory representation via modulation of hippocampus and amygdala. The overall timing of these suppression effects appear to be orchestrated by modulatory influence of BA_{10} (prefrontal area) first over rlFG then rMFG" (Depue et al., 2007). In addition to these results obtained in humans, it has been shown in animals that the increased release of an endogenous molecule (CaMKII) not only disturbs memory fixation (Wang et al., 2008), but induces the erasure of memories as well (Cao et al., 2008). Finally, the repression of unwanted memories is reinforced by sleep occurring after the experimental tasks (Rauchs et al., 2008) and this process is decreased in older people (Levy and Anderson, 2008).

Consequently, in addition to the occurrence of parapraxes, which are indices of outbursts of unconscious processes during waking, neurobiological findings can confirm the existence of unconscious repressed phenomena as postulated by Freud. For the first time, therefore, after nearly one century, his theory of a censorship process that acts during waking has been experimentally confirmed.

What Happens During the Mental Activity of Sleep, Essentially During Dreaming?

Freud, in "The interpretation of dreams" (Freud, 1900), said that the power of the censorship decreases during dreaming, allowing repressed wishes, drives, and feelings to more easily enter the sleeper's consciousness. However, he added that the true crude latent content of unconscious wishes cannot enter the dreamer's consciousness without being modified to an acceptable form by the censorship, following the primary pleasure principle; this process leads to the hallucinatory wish fulfillment. Without this transformation, the dreams would induce arousal with anxiety. According to Freud, two mechanisms are involved in the dream-work that results in the modification of the representations of the mental content: i) condensation, which is the concentration in a unique element of several ideas or feelings; and ii) displacement, which refers to "the fact that an idea's emphasis, interest or intensity is liable to be detached from it to pass on to other ideas, which were originally of little intensity but which are related to the first idea by a chain of associations" (p 121) (Laplanche and Pontalis, 2006). Another major assertion of Freud was that "the forgetting of dreams remains inexplicable unless the power of the psychical censorship is taken into account" (p 517) (Freud, 1900).

The neurobiology of dreaming is now beginning to be better known. Activation in the forebrain, particularly the cortex, is high during dreaming, as it is during waking. This was shown by the classical spontaneous EEG (Aserinsky and Kleitman, 1953, Dement, 1958, Jouvet et al., 1959), as well as by the occurrence of the gamma rhythm (Llinas and Ribary, 1993, Perez-Garci et al., 2001). The cortical activation was confirmed by the intense neuron firing (Evarts, 1964), negativity of the superficial layers as shown by their steady potential (Wurtz, 1965, Tabushi et al., 1966), increased blood pressure (Snyder et al., 1963, Kanamori et al., 1994), and increased temperature (Kawamura and Sawyer, 1965, Parmeggiani, 2007). Moreover, neuroimaging studies have also shown that the cortex is mainly activated during the dreaming sleep stage (Madsen et al., 1991, Maquet et al., 1996, Braun et al., 1997 , Nofzinger et al., 1997, Maquet et al., 2004), which has also been called rapid eye movement (REM) sleep (Dement, 1965) because of the eye movements associated with dreaming, as well as paradoxical sleep (Jouvet, 1965) because of this strong cortical activation.

Consequently, the activating processes of the forebrain during dreaming, and particularly of the cortex (which is mainly involved in mentation), are not different from waking ones. Some structures, like the associative visual cortex, the motor cortex, and the amygdala, are even more activated than they are during waking (Madsen et al., 1991, Maquet and Franck, 1997 , Braun et al., 1998, Maquet et al., 2004). Thus, it is understandable that mental activity can be generated during REM sleep.

Nevertheless, there are substantial differences between REM sleep and waking. First, while the classical EEG is similar during active waking and REM sleep, the spontaneous gamma rhythm becomes uncoupled over the cortical areas during REM sleep, unlike during waking (Perez-Garci et al., 2001 , Corsi-Cabrera et al., 2003); this also occurs between the hippocampus and the cortex (Cantero et al., 2004), and the intra-hippocampal coherence is massively decreased as well (Montgomery et al., 2008). Such disturbances of intracerebral connectivity are an index of pathological functioning that is characteristic of schizophrenia (Young et al., 1998 , Peled et al., 2000, Tononi and Edelman, 2000, Meyer-Lindenberg et al., 2001, Meyer-Lindenberg et al., 2005, Kubicki et al., 2008). Further, the spontaneous firing of cortical pyramidal neurons, contrary to the regular spiking that occurs during waking (although of similar high frequency), becomes very irregular, with high frequency bursts of discharges being interspersed with long silences (Evarts 1964). Already in the 1960s (Evarts, 1964), Evarts concluded that cortical control processes disappeared during REM sleep. Similarly, in the same period, Demetrescu et al. (Demetrescu et al., 1966) studied evoked potentials and demonstrated the presence of both activating and inhibitory influences at the cortical level during waking, with the inhibitory ones becoming minimal during REM sleep. This strong disinhibition was later confirmed by studies that also showed that the recovery cycle of cortical responsiveness is much shorter during REM sleep than during waking, a sign of disinhibition (Rossi et al., 1965, Allison, 1968). The same decrease in forebrain inhibitory processes was shown in normal individuals during REM sleep, and in schizophrenics in the waking state, through changes in the N_{100} component of the auditory evoked potential (Kisley et al., 2003).

The loss of forebrain inhibitory processes during REM sleep has also been demonstrated by data related to neurotransmitters and neuromodulators. Indeed, brainstem neurons innervating the forebrain, both noradrenergic (Hobson et al., 1975, Aston-Jones and Bloom, 1981) and serotonergic (McGinty et al., 1974 , McGinty and Harper, 1976, Rasmussen et al., 1984), become silent during REM sleep. Further, noradrenaline (Léna et al., 2005) and serotonin (Portas et al., 1998) release are minimal during REM sleep. The decreased noradrenaline in the cortex could explain the disappearance of the regular spiking seen during waking and the occurrence of the irregular bursting of neurons (Wang and McCormick, 1993). In addition, noradrenaline release is strongly decreased in the nucleus accumbens (Léna et al., 2005) and amygdala (Park, 2002). Both of these decreases are also involved in schizophrenic disease, since inhibitors of noradrenergic (Friedman et al., 1999, Linner et al., 2002) and serotonergic (Silver et al., 2000, Van Hes et al., 2003) transporters (uptake inhibitors) are now included in new treatments for schizophrenia.

Dopamine, the neurons of which continue to fire during REM sleep (Miller et al., 1983 , Trulson and Preussler, 1984, Dahan et al., 2007), is also decreased in the prefrontal cortex during REM sleep, whereas it is maximal in the nucleus accumbens (Léna et al., 2005). This latter release is related to the REM-sleep-associated bursting mode of dopaminergic neuron firing (Gonon, 1988 , Grace, 1991, Suaud-Chagny et al., 1992 , Schultz, 2007) in the mesolimbic tract (Miller et al., 1983, Dahan et al., 2007). The decreased dopamine release in the prefrontal cortex could be involved in the decreased self-awareness and control of cognitive functions that is encountered both during REM sleep and in schizophrenia. (Okubo et al., 1997, Abi-Dargham and Moore, 2003). In any case, dopamine in the prefrontal cortex is crucial for dreaming, since dreaming is suppressed after surgical leukotomy (Solms, 2000). In contrast, the maximal release observed in the nucleus accumbens could be responsible for vivid dreaming, as observed with dopaminergic agonists (Larsen and Tandberg, 2001, Perry and Piggott, 2003), and for the psychotic-like mentation seen during dreaming. Indeed, excess dopamine has long been evidenced in the nucleus accumbens in schizophrenia (MacKay et al., 1982), and neuroleptics both decrease dreaming and improve schizophrenic symptoms (Solms, 2000 , Jakovljevic et al., 2003).

There are also clear similarities with respect to glutamate release in the prefrontal cortex and the nucleus accumbens during dreaming and in schizophrenia. Indeed, the release is unchanged in both cases (Lauriat et al., 2005, Léna et al., 2005) in the prefrontal cortex, while it is strongly decreased in the nucleus accumbens (Léna et al., 2005), promoting both vivid dreaming (Reeves et al., 2001) and psychotic symptoms (Grace, 2000, Heresco-Levy, 2000).

Finally, acetylcholine, which is crucial for cognitive processes (Perry et al., 1999, Sarter and Bruno, 2000), is also decreased in the cortex during dreaming when compared to its active waking level (Marrosu et al., 1995). This decrease promotes schizophrenic hallucinations (Collerton et al., 2005) as well as, highly probably, dreaming ones.

One question remains open: the function of GABA. Schizophrenics show a prefrontal deficit in GABA in the prefrontal cortex (Lewis, 2000, Lewis et al., 2005). Since the corresponding interneurons are innervated by dopaminergic terminals, and there is a dopaminergic deficit in the prefrontal cortex during REM sleep (Léna et al., 2005), it is possible that there is a parallel deficit in prefrontal GABA during REM sleep. However, this has not been demonstrated to date.

Neuroimaging studies have also revealed disturbances in forebrain functioning during REM sleep and have uncovered strong similarities between dreaming and schizophrenia.

First, the dorsolateral prefrontal cortex is deactivated during REM sleep (Maquet et al., 1996, Braun et al., 1997 , Maquet et al., 2004) as well as in schizophrenia, particularly when cognitive processes are impaired (Weinberger et al., 1986, Berman et al., 1993 , Fletcher et al., 1998). This deactivation was first shown by a decrease in glucose uptake (Buschbaum et al., 1982). Moreover, the primary visual cortex has been shown to be deactivated during REM sleep, with the associative visual cortex being strongly activated (Braun et al., 1998); this result has been questioned, however (Hong et al., 2008). This deactivation could reflect a sensory disconnection that is reinforced at the thalamic level by a depolarization (inhibition) of presynaptic afferents (Dagnino et al., 1969, Ghelarducci et al., 1970, Steriade, 1970, Gandolfo et al., 1980). This disconnection is also evidenced during REM sleep by the non-resetting of the gamma rhythm by sensory stimulation (Llinas and Ribary, 1993). Such global sensory deprivation is now known to promote hallucinations (Behrendt and Young, 2005) due to the failure of sensory constraints as observed both during dreaming and in schizophrenia. This disconnection from sensory inputs could also explain the increased pain threshold observed during psychotic episodes (Griffin and Tyrrell, 2003). Finally, concerning the cognitive perception of the sensory gating control, there is a failure in the differentiation between self- and external stimulation (tickle) at the outcome of REM sleep dreaming, as there is in schizophrenia (Blagrove et al., 2006)

A final neuroimaging-related result concerns the posterior cingulate cortex. It must be mentioned that the dorsolateral prefrontal cortex and the posterior cingulate cortex, both of which are deactivated during REM sleep (Maquet et al., 1996, Maquet et al., 2004), are also deactivated when piano concertists are so involved in their playing that they "lose themselves" (Parsons et al., 2005) and are thus somewhat disconnected from the environment, as is the case in schizophrenia (Gottesmann, 2006a, Gottesmann, 2007).

DISCUSSION

Based on the above-presented results, it appears that, with the exception of parapraxes--indices of unconscious contents bursting into waking consciousness--unwanted memories can be rejected from consciousness. Accordingly, a censorship process acts to prevent emotional mental contents from disturbing behavioral adaptation. These conclusions are in accordance with Freud's repression model, making this the first time that the quasi-closed dogma of psychoanalytic theory has found clear-cut neurobiological confirmation.

These results concern the processes that occur during waking. With respect to the dreaming sleep stage (REM sleep), current experimental results are less clear. Indeed, Hobson and colleagues (Hobson et al., 1998) carefully described the characteristics of dreaming, which includes "sensory hallucinations, bizarre imagery...diminished self-awareness, orientational instability... intensification of emotion, instinctual behaviors" (p R2). These properties of dreaming resemble the psychological disturbances encountered in the psychotic disease of schizophrenia. As shown in the previous paragraphs, today's neurobiological findings have uncovered numerous similarities between dreaming and schizophrenia. In fact, these modern experimental results have confirmed old assertions of philosophers ("the madman is a waking dreamer" Kant in (Freud, 1900)), writers ("dream is a kind of delirium" (Maury, 1861)) and neuropsychiatrists (" it is obvious that dream and madness spurt out from the same source" (Ey, 1967)), who concluded long ago that brain functioning during the dreaming sleep stage is strongly disturbed.

Freud's theory holds that active cognitive processes persist during the REM sleep dreaming stage, and that a dream-work process, directed by a censorship mechanism, transforms unconscious feelings and wishes into acceptable forms so that they can enter the sleeper's consciousness as mainly visual symbolic representations, without inducing disturbances that would lead to arousal. There is here a small contradiction with Freud's own assertion that, because of attenuated censorship, forbidden contents could enter the dreamer's consciousness. Neurobiological results show that the different brain structures are not only disconnected from one another, but that there is a strong decrease in the central inhibitory processes (as shown by electrophysiological, neurochemical and neuroimaging results) that control the activating ones during waking. Amid such disturbed brain functioning, it would be rather unexpected to find advanced cognitive processes. In fact, "there is more censorship in the waking analysis of dreams than during the dream itself" (p 17) (Blechner, 2006)

Consequently, while the hyper-associative nature of dreaming content (Hobson and Pace-Schott, 1999) can seemingly give rise to certain transient, organized content--so that it can be said that "an uninterpreted dream is like an unread letter" (Talmud)--most often the mental content of dreaming involves a psychotic-like activity.

The other main assertion of Freud concerns the immediate or rapid forgetting of dreams. Here also, because of the numerous disturbances of forebrain functioning that take place during REM sleep, it is difficult to retain the existence of a censorship mechanism which, like the "mystic writing-pad" (Freud, 1925), would erase the memory of dreams because of repression phenomena. There are, however, neurobiological data which are able to explain this forgetting. First, cortisol, which impairs memory processes (Kirschbaum et al., 1996, Payne and Nadel, 2004), is mainly released in the early morning, just prior to morning arousal, when the main REM sleep phase occurs. In addition, noradrenaline release reappears in the few seconds preceding arousal (Aston-Jones and Bloom, 1981). This neuromodulator is involved in higher integrated cognitive processes (Arnsten and Li, 2005, Berridge et al., 2006 , Milstein et al., 2007), and its reappearance certainly participates in the recovery of waking functions and disrupts previous REM sleep processes. Further, the prefrontal cortex has highly important functions in memory processes. Its recovery of functioning upon arousal (Balkin et al., 2002) could prevent the recording of dreams into waking memory. Finally, a possible burst of endogenous CaMKII (Cao et al., 2008 , Wang et al., 2008) release upon the reappearance of noradrenaline prior to awakening could explain the evanescence of dreams.

To conclude, for the first time, neurobiology is in the position to confirm one of the main assertions of psychoanalytic theory, i.e. the existence of unconscious phenomena during waking, namely the repression of unwanted memories which are prevented from accessing consciousness. These results confirm and underscore Freud's old description of the bursting-out of unconscious phenomena as evidenced by parapraxes. The censorship responsible for these repression processes is more obvious during waking than during dreaming, in REM sleep. Indeed, the forebrain, which is responsible for mentation, is so disturbed during this sleep stage that it is difficult to find objective criteria of advanced cognitive processes that could support a hypothetical dream-work generated by a censorship process (Gottesmann, 2006b).

Acknowledgment

I thank Dr. Peter Follette for his attentive improvement of the English.

References

Abi-Dargham, A. and Moore, H., 2003. Prefrontal DA transmission at D1 receptors and the pathology of schizophrenia. *Neuroscientist.* 9, 404-416.

Allison, T., 1968. Recovery cycles of primary evoked potentials in cats sensorimotor cortex. Experentia. 24, 240-241.

Anderson, M. C. and Green, C., 2001. Suppressing unwanted memories by exceutive control. *Nature.* 410, 366-369.

Anderson, M. C., Ochsner, K. N., Kuhl, B., Cooper, J., Robertson, E., Gabrielli, S. W., Glover, G. H. and Gabrielli, J. D. E., 2004. Neural systems underlying the suppression of unwanted memories. *Science.* 303, 232-235.

Arnsten, A. F. and Li, B. M., 2005. Neurobiology of executive functions: catecholamine influences on prefrontal cortical functions. *Biol. Psychiat.* 57, 1377-1384.

Aserinsky, E. and Kleitman, N., 1953. Regularly occurring periods of eye motility, and concomitant phenomena during sleep. *Science.* 118, 273-274.

Aston-Jones, G. and Bloom, F. E., 1981. Activity of norepinephrine-containing neurons in behaving rats anticipates fluctuations in the sleep-waking cycle. *J. Neurosci.* 1, 876-886.

Balkin, T. J., Braun, A. R., Wesensten, N. J., Jeffries, K., Varga, M., Baldwin, P., Belenky, G. and Herscovitch, P., 2002. The process of awakening: a PET study of regional brain activity patterns mediating the re-establishment of alertness and consciousness. *Brain.* 125, 2308-2319.

Behrendt, R. P. and Young, C., 2005. Hallucinations in schizophrenia, sensori impairment and brain disease: an unified model. *Behav. Brain Sci.* 27, 771-787.

Berger, H., 1929. Ueber das electroenkephalogram des Menschen. *Arch Psychiat Nervenkrank.* 87, 527-570.

Berman, K. F., Doran, A. R., Pickar, D. and Weinberger, D. R., 1993. Is the mechanism of prefrontal hypofunction in depression the same as in schizophrenia? Regional cerebral blood flow during cognitive activation. *Br .J. Psychiat.* 162, 183-192.

Berridge, C. W., Devilbiss, D. M., Andrzejewski, M. E., Arnsten, A. F., Kelley, A. E., Schmeichel, B., Hamilton, C. and Spencer, R. C., 2006. Methylphenidate preferentially increases catecholamine neurotransmission within the prefrontal cortex at low doses that enhance cognitive function. *Biol. Psychiat.* 60, 1111-1120.

Blagrove, M., Blakemore, S. J. and Thayer, B. R. J., 2006. The ability to self-tickle following rapid eye movement sleep dreaming. Conscious Cogn. 15, 285-294.

Blechner, M. J., 2006. A post-Freudian psychoanalytic model of dreaming. *Neuro-Psychoanal.* 8, 17-20.

Bouyer, J. J., Montaron, M. F. and Rougeul, A., 1981. Fast fronto-parietal rhythms during combined focused attentive behavior and immobility in cat: cortical and thalamic localizations. *Electroenceph. Clin. Neurophysiol.* 51, 244-252.

Braun, A. R., Balkin, T. J., Wesensten, N. J., Carson, R. E., Varga, M., Baldwin, P., Selbie, S., Belenky, G. and Herscovitch, P., 1997. Regional cerebral blood flow throughout the sleep-wake cycle: An ^{15}0 PET study. *Brain.* 120, 1173-1197.

Braun, A. R., Balkin, T. J., Wesensten, N. J., Gwardry, f., Carson, R. E., Varga, M., Baldwin, P., Belenky, G. and Herscovitch, P., 1998. Dissociated pattern of activity in visual cortices and their projections during human rapid eye movement sleep. *Science.* 279, 91-95.

Bremer, F., 1935. Cerveau "isolé" et physiologie du sommeil. C R Soc Biol. 118, 1235-1241.

Bremer, F., 1936. Nouvelles recherches sur le mécanisme du sommeil. *C R Soc. Biol.* 122, 460-464.

Bubnoff, N. and Heidenhain, R., 1881. Ueber Erregungs-Hemmungsvorgänge innerhalb der motorischen Hirncentren. In: Pflüger EFW (Ed*). Arch. Gesam. Physiol.*, pp 137-202.

Buschbaum, M. S., Ingvar, D. H., Kessler, R., Waters, R. N., Cappelletti, J., Van Kammen, D. P., King, A. C., Johnson, J. L., Manning, R. G., Flynn, R. W., Bunney, W. E. J. and Sokoloff, L., 1982. Cerebral glucography with positron tomography, use in normal subjects and in patients with schizophrenia. *Arch. Gen. Psychiat.* 39, 251-259.

Cantero, J. L., Atienza, M., Madsen, J. R. and Stickgold, R., 2004. Gamma EEG dynamics in neocortex and hippocampus during human wakefulness and sleep. *Neuroimage.* 22, 1271-1280.

Cao, X., Wang, H., Mei, B., An, S., Yin, L., Wang, L. P. and Tsien, J., 2008. Indicible and selective erasure of memories in the mouse brain via chemical-genetic manipulation. Neuron. 60, 353-366.

Collerton, D., Perry, E. and McKeith, I., 2005. A novel perception and attention deficit model for recurrent visual hallucinations. *Brain Behav. Sci.* 28, 737-757.

Corsi-Cabrera, M., Miro, E., del Rio Portilla, Y., Perez-Garci, E., Villanueva, Y. and Guevera, M., 2003. Rapid eye movement sleep dreaming is characterized by uncoupled EEG activity netween frontal abd perceptual cortical regions. *Brain Cogn.* 51, 337-345.

Creutzfeldt, O., Baumgartner, G. and Schoen, L., 1956. Reaktionen einzelner Neurons des senso-motorischen cortex nach elektrischen Reizen. I Hemmung und Erregung nach direkten und contralateralen Einzelreizen. *Arch. Psychiat Nervenkrank.* 194, 597-619.

Dagnino, N., Favale, E., Loeb, C., Manfredi, M. and Seitun, A., 1969. Presynaptic and postsynaptic changes in specific thalamic nuclei during deep sleep. *Arch. Ital. Biol.* 107, 668-684.

Dahan, L., Astier, B., Vautrelle, N., Urbain, N., Kocsis, B. and Chouvet, G., 2007. Prominent burst firing of dopaminergic neurons in the vental tegmental area during paradoxical sleep. *Neuropschopharmacology.* 32, 1232-1241.

Dement, W. C., 1958. The occurrence of low voltage fast electroencephalogram patterns during behavioral sleep in the cat. *Electroenceph. Clin. Neurophysiol.* 10, 291-296.

Dement, W. C., 1965. Recent studies on the biological role of rapid eye movement sleep. *Am. J. Psychiat.* 122, 404-408.

Demetrescu, M., Demetrescu, M. and Iosif, G., 1966. Diffuse regulation of visual thalamo-cortical responsiveness during sleep and wakefulness. *Electroenceph. Clin. Neurophysiol.* 20, 450-469.

Depue, B. E., Banich, M. T. and Curran, T., 2006. Suppression of emotional and nonemotional content in memory. *Psychol. Sci.* 17, 441-447.

Depue, B. E., Curran, T. and Banich, M. T., 2007. Prefrontal regions orchestrate suppression of emotional memories via a two-phase process. *Science.* 317, 215-219.

Evarts, E. V., 1964. Temporal patterns of discharge of pyramidal tract neurons during sleep and waking in the monkey. *J. Neurophysiol.* 27, 152-171.

Ey, H., 1967. La dissolution du champ de la conscience dans le phénomène sommeil-veille et ses rapports avec la psychopathologie. *Pres. Med.* 75, 575-578.

Fechner, G. T., 1848. Über das Lustprinzip des Handels. Zeitschrift für Philososphie und Philosophische Kritik, 11(quoted by Laplache and Pontalis p 322 and 325 and Gottesmann, C. 1967 thesis p 1113).

Fletcher, P. C., McKenna, P. J., Frith, C. D., Grasby, P. M., Friston, K. J. and Dolan, R. J., 1998. Brain activation in schizophrenia during a graded memory task studied with functional neuroimaging. *Arch. Gen. Psychiat.* 55, 1001-1008.

Foote, S. L., Freedman, R. and Oliver, A. P., 1975. Effects of putative neurotransmitters on neuronal activity on monkey auditory cortex. *Brain Res.* 86, 229-242.

Freud, S., 1897. Letter to Wilhem Fliess (22 december). In: Bonaparte, M. (Ed.), La naissance de la Psychanalyse. Presses Universitaires de France, Paris, pp. 211-213.

Freud, S., 1900. The interpretation of dreams. The Hogart Press,, London.

Freud, S., 1901. The psychopathology of everyday life. In: Edition, S. (Ed.), vol.VI, London.

Freud, S., 1925. A note upon the " mystic writing-pad". Standart Edition, vol 19. pp 227-232., The Hogart Press, London, 1955.

Friedman, J. I., Adler, D. N. and Davis, K. L., 1999. The role of norepinephrine in the physiopathology of cognitive disorders: potential applications to the treatment of cognitive dysfunction in schizophrenia and Alzheimer's disease. *Biol .Psychiat.* 46, 1243-1252.

Gandolfo, G., Arnaud, C. and Gottesmann, C., 1980. Transmission in the ventrobasal complex of rat during the sleep-waking cycle. *Brain Res. Bull.* 5, 921-927.

Ghelarducci, B., Pisa, M. and Pompeiano, M., 1970. Transformation of somatic afferent volleys across the prethalamic and thalamic components of the lemniscal sytem during the rapid eye movements of sleep. *Electroenceph Clin. Neurophysiol.* 29, 348-357.

Gonon, F. G., 1988. Nonlinear relationship between impulse flow and dopamine released by rat midbrain dopaminergic neurons as studied by in vivo electrochemistry. *Neuroscience.* 24, 19-28.

Gottesmann, C., 1967. Recherche sur la psychophysiologie du sommeil chez le Rat. Presses du Palais Royal, Paris (still available, discussion and summary in English).

Gottesmann, C., 1970. La psychophysiologie du sommeil. *Bull. Psychol.* 24, 520-528.

Gottesmann, C., 1971. Psychophysiologie du sommeil. *Ann. Psychol.* 71, 451-488.

Gottesmann, C., 1999. Neurophysiological support of consciousness during waking and sleep. *Prog. Neurobiol.* 59, 469-508.

Gottesmann, C., 2006a. The dreaming sleep stage: a new neurobiological model of schizophrenia? *Neuroscience.* 140, 1105-1115.

Gottesmann, C., 2006b. Neurobiological disturbances during the dreaming-sleep stage can explain dream bizarreness without recourse to censorship. *Neuro-Psychoanalysis.* 8, 27-32.

Gottesmann, C., 2007. A neurobiological history of dreaming. In: McNamara, P. and Barrett, D. (Eds.), The Science of Dreaming, vol.1. Greenwood Publishers, Westport, pp. 1-51.

Grace, A. A., 1991. Phasic versus tonic dopamine release and the modulation of dopamine system responsivity: a hypothesis for the etiology of schizophrenia. *Neuroscience.* 41, 1-24.

Grace, A. A., 2000. Gating information flow within the limbic system and the pathophysiology of schizophrenia. *Brain Res. Rev.* 31, 330-341.

Griffin, J. and Tyrrell, I., 2003. Human Givens: A new approach to emotional health and clear thinking. HG Publishing., New York.

Helmholtz, H. v., 1860. Handbuch der physiologischen Optik ('unconscious conclusions', p 601, quoted by Pavlov, I. : Oeuvres Choisies p 225), Leipzig.

Heresco-Levy, U., 2000. N-methyl-D-aspartate (NMDA) receptor-based treatment approaches in schizophrenia: the first decade. *Int J. Neuropharmacol.* 3, 243-258.

Hobson, J. A., McCarley, R. W. and Wyzinski, P. W., 1975. Sleep cycle oscillation: reciprocal discharge by two brainstem neuronal groups. *Science.* 189, 55-58.

Hobson, J. A. and Pace-Schott, E., 1999. Response to commentaries. *Neuro-Pasychoanalysis.* 1, 206-224.

Hobson, J. A., Stickgold, R. and Pace-Schott, E. F., 1998. The neuropsychology of REM sleep dreaming. *NeuroReport.* 9, R1-R14.

Hong, C. C. H., Harris, J. C., Pearlson, G. D., Kim, J.-S., Calhoun, V. C., Fallon, J. H., Golay, X., Gillen, J. S., Simmonds, D. J., van Zijl, P. C. M., Zee, D. S. and Pekar, J. J., 2008. fMRI evidence for multisensory recruitment associated with rapid eye movements during sleep. *Hum. Brain Map.* In press.

Jakovljevic, M., Sagud, M. and Mihaljevic-Peles, A., 2003. Olanzapine in the treatment-resistant,combat-related PTSD- a series of case reports. *Acta Psychiat. Scand.* 107, 394-396.

Jouvet, M., 1965. Paradoxical sleep: a study of its nature and mechanisms. In: Akert, K. B., C.Schadé J.P. (eds) (Ed.), Sleep mechanisms, vol.18. *Progress in Brain Research,* pp. 20-62.

Jouvet, M., Michel, F. and Courjon, J., 1959. Sur un stade d'activité électrique rapide au cours du sommeil physiologique. *C R Soc. Biol.* 153, 1024-1028.

Kanamori, N., Sakai, K., Sei, H., Salvert, D., Vanni-Mercier, G., Yamamoto, M. and Jouvet, M., 1994. Power spectral analysis of blood pressure fluctuations during sleep in normal and decerebrate cats. *Arch. Ital. Biol.* 132, 105-115.

Kandel, E. R., 1999. Biology and the future of psychoanalysis: a new intellectual framework for psychiatry revisited. *Am. J. Psychiat.* 156, 505-524.

Kawamura, H. and Sawyer, C. H., 1965. Elevation in brain temperature during paradoxical sleep. *Science.* 150, 912-913.

Kirschbaum, C., Wolf, O. T., May, M., Wippich, W. and Hellhammer, D. H., 1996. Stress- and treatment-induced elevations of cortisol levels associated with impaired declarative memory in healthy adults. *Life Sci.* 58, 1475-1483.

Kisley, M. A., Olincy A., Robbins E., Polk S.D., Adler L.E., Waldo M.C. and Freedman, R., 2003. Sensory gating impairement associated with schizophrenia persists into REM sleep;. *Psychophysiology.* 40, 29-38.

Krnjevic, K. and Phillis, J. W., 1963. Actions of certain amines on cerebral cortex neurons. *Brit J. Pharmacol.* 20, 471-490.

Krnjevic, K., Randic, M. and Straughan, D. W., 1966. Pharmacology of cortical inhibition. *J. Physiol.* London. 184, 78-105.

Kubicki, M., Styner, M., Gerig, G., Markant, D., Smith, K., MacCarley, R. W. and Shenton, M. E., 2008. Reduced interhemispheric connectivity in schizophrenic-tractography based segmentation of the corpus callosum. *Schizophr .Res.* 106, 125-131.

Laplanche, J. and Pontalis, J. B., 2006. The language of psychoanalysis. Karnac Books, London.

Larsen, J. P. and Tandberg, E., 2001. Sleep disorders with Parkinson's disease: epidemiology and management. *CNS Drugs*. 15, 267-275.

Lauriat, T. L., Dracheva, S., Chin, B., Schmeidler, J., McInnes, L. A. and Haroutunian, V., 2005. Quantitative analysis of glutamate transporter mRNA expression in prefrontal and primary visual cortex in normal and schizophrenic brain. *Neuroscience.* 137, 843-851.

Léna, I., Parrot, S., Deschaux, O., Muffat, S., Sauvinet, V., Renaud, B., Suaud-Chagny, M. F. and Gottesmann, C., 2005. Variations in the extracellular levels of dopamine, noradrenaline, glutamate and aspartate across the sleep-wake cycle in the medial prefrontal cortex and nucleus accumbens of freely moving rats. *J. Neurosci. Res.* 81, 891-899.

Levy, B. J. and Anderson, M. C., 2008. Individual differences in the suppression of unwanted memories: The executive deficit hypothesis. *Acta Psychologica*. 127, 623)535.

Lewis, D. A., 2000. GABAergic local circuit neurons and prefrontal cortical dysfunction in schizophrenia. *Brain Res. Rev*. 31, 270-276.

Lewis, D. A., Hashimoto, T. and Volk, D. W., 2005. Cortical inhibitory neurons in schizophrenia. *Nat. Rev. Neurosci.* 6, 312-324.

Linner, L., Wiker, C., Wadenberg, M. L., Schalling, M. and Svensson, T. H., 2002. Noradrenaline reuptake inhibition enhances the antipsychotic-like effect of raclopride and potentiates D2-blockade-induced dopamine release in the medial prefrontal cortex of the rat. *Neuropsychpharmacology*. 27, 691-698.

Llinas, R. and Ribary, U., 1993. Coherent 40 Hz oscillation characterizes dream state in humans. *Proc Nat Acad Sci USA,*. 90, 2078-2081.

MacKay, A. V., Iversen, L. L., Rossor, M., Spokes, E., Bird, E., Arregui, A. and Snyder, S., 1982. Increased brain dopamine and dopamine receptors in schizophrenia. *Arch. Gen. Psychiat.* 39, 991-997.

Madsen, P. L., Holm, S., Vorstrup, S., Friberg, L., Lassen, N. A. and Wildschiodtz, G., 1991. Human regional cerebral blood flow during rapid-eye-movement sleep. *J. Cerbr. Blood* Flow Met. 11, 502-507.

Maquet, P. and Franck, G., 1997. REM sleep and amygdala. *Mol. Psychiat.* 2, 195-196.

Maquet, P., Peters, J. M., Aerts, J., Delfiore, G., Degueldre, C. and Luxen, A., Franck, G.,, 1996. Functional neuroanatomy of human rapid-eye-movement sleep and dreaming. *Nature.* 383, 163-166.

Maquet, P., Ruby, P., Schw artz, S., Laurey, S., Albouy, T., Dang-Vu, T., Desseilles, M., Boly, M., Melchior, G. and Peigneux, P., 2004. Regional organisation of brain activity during paradoxical sleep. *Arch. Ital. Biol.* 142, 413-419.

Marrosu, F., Portas, C., Mascia, M. F., Casu, M. A., Fa, M., Giagheddu, M., Imperato, A. and gessa, G. L., 1995. Microdialysis measurement of cortical and hippocampal acetylcholine release during sleep-wake cycle in freely moving cats. *Brain Res.* 671, 329-332.

Maury, F., 1861. Le sommeil et les rêves. Didier (ed), 156.

McCormick, D. A., Wang, Z. and Huguenard, J., 1993. Neurotransmitter control of neocortical neuronal activity and excitability. *Cereb. Cort.* 3, 387-398.

McGinty, D. J. and Harper, R. M., 1976. Dorsal raphe neurons: depression of firing during sleep in cats. *Brain Res.* 101, 569-575.

McGinty, D. J., Harper, R. M. and Fairbanks, M. K., 1974. Neuronal unit activity and the control of sleep states. In: Weitzman, E. D. (Ed.), In: Advances in Sleep Research, Vol 1. Spectrum, New York, pp. 173-216.

Meyer-Lindenberg, A., Olsen, R. K., Kohn, P. D., Brown, T., Egan, M. F., Weinberber, D. R. and Berman, K. F., 2005. Regionally specific disturbance of dorsolateral prefrontal-hippocampal function connectivity in schizophrenia. *Arch. Gen. Psychiat.* 62, 379-386.

Meyer-Lindenberg, A., Poline, J. B., Kohn, P. D., Holt, J. L., Egan, M. F., Weinberger, D. R. and Berman, K. F., 2001. Evidence for abnormal cortical functional connectivity during working memory in schizophrenia. *Am. J. Psychiat.* 158, 1809-1817.

Miller, J. D., Farber, J., Gatz, P., Roffwarg, H. and German, D., 1983. Activity of mesencephalic dopamine and non-dopamine neurons across stages of sleep and waking in the rat. *Brain Res.* 273, 133-141.

Milstein, J. A., Lehmann, O., Theobald, D. E., Dalley, J. W. and Robbins, E., 2007. Selective depletion of cortical noradrenaline by ant-domaine beta-hydroxylase-saporin impairs attentional function and enhances the effect of guafacine in the rat. *Psychophamacology.* 190, 51-63.

Montgomery, S. M., Sirota, A. and Buzsaki, G., 2008. Theta and gamma coordination of hippocampal networks during waking and rapid eye movement sleep. *J. Neurosci.* 28, 6731-6741.

Moruzzi, G. and Magoun, H. W., 1949. Brain stem reticular formation and activation of the EEG. *Electroenceph Clin. Neurophysiol.* 1, 455-473.

Nofzinger, E. A., Mintun, M. A., Wiseman, M. B. and Kupfer, J., 1997. Forebrain activation during REM sleep: an FDG PET study. *Brain Res.* 770, 192-201.

Okubo, Y., Suhara, T., Kobahashi, K., Inoue, O., Terasaki, O., Someya, Y., Sassa, T., Sudo, Y., Matsushima, E., Iyo, M., Tateno, Y. and TOru, M., 1997. Decreased prefrontal dopamine D1 receptors in schizophrenia revealed by PET. *Nature.* 385, 634-636.

Park, S. P., 2002. In vovo microdialysis measures of extracellular norepinephrine in the rat amygdala during sleep-wakefulness. *J. Korean Med. Sci.* 17, 395-399.

Parmeggiani, P. L., 2007. REM sleep related increase in brain temperature: a physiologic problem. *Arch. Ital. Biol.* 145, 13-21.

Parsons, L. M., Sergent, J., Hodges, D. A. and Fox, P. T., 2005. The brain basis of piano performance. *Neuropsychologia.* 43, 199-215.

Payne, J. L. and Nadel, L., 2004. Sleep, dreaming and memory consolidation: the role of the stress hormone cortisol. Learn Mem. 11, 671-678.

Peled, A., Geva, A. B., Kremen, W. S., Blankfeld, H. M., Esfandiarfard, R. and Nordahl, T. E., 2000. Functional connectivity and working memory in schizophrenia: an EEG study. *Int. J. Neurosci.* 106, 47-61.

Perez-Garci, E., del Rio-Portilla, Y., Guevara, M. A., Arce, C. and Corsi-cabrera, M., 2001. Paradoxical sleep is characterized by uncoupled gamma activity between frontal and perceptual cortical regions. *Sleep.* 24, 118-126.

Perry, E., Walker, M., Grace, J. and Perry, R., 1999. Acetylcholine in mind: a neurotransmitter of consciousness? *Trends in Neuroscience.* 22, 273-280.

Perry, E. K. and Piggott, 2003. Neurotransmitter mechanisms of dreaming: implication of modulatory systems based on dream intensity. In: Pace-Schott, E. et al. (Eds.), Sleep and dreaming. Scientific advances and reconsiderations. Cambridge University Press, Cambridge, pp. 202-204.

Portas, C., Bjorvatn, B., Fagerland, S., Gronli, J., Mundal, V., Sorensen, E. and Ursin, R., 1998. On-line detection of extracellular levels of serotonin in dorsal raphe nucleus and frontal cortex over the sleep/wake cycle in the freely moving rat. *Neuroscience.* 83, 807-814.

Rasmussen, K., Heym, J. and Jacobs, B. L., 1984. Activity of serotonin-containing neurons in nucleus centralis superior of freely moving cats. *Exp. Neurol.* 83, 302-317.

Rauchs, G., Feyers, D., Maquet, P. and Collette, F., 2008. Does sleep favour forgetting of irrelevant information. *J. Sleep Res.* 17 (suppl.1), 10.

Reader, T. A., Ferron, A., Descarries, L. and Jasper, H. H., 1979. Modulatory role for biogenic amines in the cerebral cortex. Microiontopheric studies. *Brain Res.* 160, 219-229.

Reeves, M., Lindholm, D. E., Myles, P. S., Fletcher, H. and Hunt, J. O., 2001. Adding ketamine to morphine for patient-controlled analgesia after major abdominal surgery: a double-blind, randomized trial. *Anesth. Analg.* 93, 116-120.

Ribary, U., Ionnides, A. A., Singh, K. D., Hasson, R., Bolton, J., Lado, F., Mogilner, A. and Llinas, R., 1991. Magnetic field tomography of coherent thalamocortical 40 Hz oscillations in humans. *Proc. Nat. Acad. Sci USA*,. 88, 11037-11041.

Rossi, G. F., Palestini, M., Pisano, M. and Rosadini, G., 1965. An experimental study of the cortical reactivity during sleep and wakefulness. In : Aspects anatomo-fonctionnels de la physiologie du sommeil. CNRS, Paris,, pp 509-532.

Sarter, M. and Bruno, J. P., 2000. Cortical cholinergic inputs mediating arousal, attentional processing and dreaming: differential afferent regulation of the basal forebrain by telencephalic and brainstem afferents. *Neuroscience.* 95, 933-952.

Schultz, W., 2007. Multiple dopamine functions at different time course. *Ann. Rev. Neurosci.* 20, 259-288.

Silver, H., Barash, I., Aharon, N., Kaplan, A. and Poyurovsky, M., 2000. Fluvoxamine augmentation of antipsychotics improves negative symptoms in psychotic chronic schizophrenic patients: a placebo-controlled study. *Int. Clin. Psychopharmacol.* 15, 257-261.

Snyder, F., Hobson, J. A. and Goldfrank, F., 1963. Blood pressure changes during human sleep. *Science.* 142, 1313-1314.

Solms, M., 2000. Dreaming and REM sleep are controlled by different brain mechanisms. *Behav. Brain Sci.* 23, 843-850.

Steriade, M., 1970. Ascending control of thalamic and cortical responsiveness. *Int Rev. Neurobiol.* 12, 87-144.

Steriade, M., 1996. Arousal: revisiting the reticular system. *Science.* 272, 225-226.

Steriade, M., Amzica, F. and Contreras, D., 1996. Synchronization of fast (30-40 Hz) spontaneous cortical rhythms during brain activation. *J. Neurosci.* 16, 392-417.

Suaud-Chagny, M. F., Chergui, K., Chouvet, G. and Gonon, F., 1992. Relationship between dopamine release in the rat nucleus accumbens and the decharge activity of dopaminergic neurons during local in vivo application of amin acids in the ventral tegmental area. *Neuroscience*. 49, 63-72.

Tabushi, K., Hishikawa, Y., Ueyama, M. and Kaneko, Z., 1966. Cortical D.C. potential changes associated with spontaneous sleep in the cat. *Arch. Ital. Biol.* 104, 152-162.

Tononi, G. and Edelman, G. M., 2000. Schizophrenia and the mechanism of conscious integration. *Brain Res. Rev.* 31, 391-400.

Trulson, M. E. and Preussler, D. W., 1984. Dopamine-containing ventral tegmental area neurons in freely moving cats: activity during the sleep-waking cycle and effects of stress. *Exp. Neurol.* 83, 367-377.

Van Hes, R., Smid, P., Stroomer, C. N., Tipker, K., Tulp, M. T., Van der Heyden, J. A., McCreary, A. C., Hesselink, M. B. and Kruse, C. G., 2003. SL V310, a novel, potential antipsychotic, combining potent dopamine d2 receptor antagonism with serotonin reuptake inhibition. *Bioorg. Med. Chem. Lett.* 13, 405-408.

Wang, H., Feng, R., Wang, L. P., Li, F., Cao, X. and Tsien, J., 2008. CAMKII activation state underlies synaptic labile phase of LTP and short-term memory formation. *Curr. Biol.* 18, 1546-1554.

Wang, Z. and McCormick, D. A., 1993. Control of firing mode of corticotectal and corticopontine layer V burst-generating neurons by norepinephrine, acetylcholine and 1S, 3R-ACPD. *J. Neurosci.* 13, 2199-2216.

Weinberger, D. R., Berman, K. F. and Zec, R.F.,, 1986. Physiological dysfunction of dorsolateral prefrontal cortex in schizophrenia. 1. Regional cerebral blood flow evidence. *Arch. Gen. Psychiat.* 43, 114-124.

Wurtz, R. H., 1965. Steady potential shifts in the rat during desynchronized sleep. *Electroenceph. Clin.-Neurophysiol.* 19, 521-523.

Young, C. E., Beach, T. G., Falkai, P. and Honer, W. G., 1998. SNAP-25 deficit and hippocampal connectivity in schizophrenia. *Cer. Cort.* 8, 261-268.

In: Psychiatric Research Trends: Dreams and Geriatric Psychiatry ISBN 978-1-60741-760-6
Editors: Daniella M. Montez, pp.117-131

Chapter 7

RECENT ADVANCES IN ECOLOGICAL STUDIES OF ELDERLY SUICIDES: COMMENTARY

Ajit Shah[1]
Professor of Ageing, Ethnicity and Mental Health, International School for Communities, Rights and Inclusion, University of Central Lancashire, Preston, United Kingdom and Consultant Psychiatrist, West London Mental Health NHS Trust, London, United Kingdom

INTRODUCTION

The elderly population size is increasing due to prolonged life expectancy and falling birth rates worldwide (Shah and McKenzie, 2007). Traditionally, suicide rates increased with ageing. A recent cross-national study of 62 developing and developed countries reported an increase in suicide rates with ageing in males and females in 25 and 27 countries respectively (Shah, 2007a). Thus, suicides in the elderly are an important public health concern. Comprehensive understanding of the substantial worldwide variation in population patterns of suicide may be critical for developing prevention programmes (Knox et al., 2004). While much is known about individual level risk factors (e.g. Conwell et al., 1991; Catell and Jolley, 1995; Harwood et al., 2001), this strategy has limitations in unmasking more distal causes of suicide (Rehkopf and Buka, 2006). Moreover, detailed knowledge of distal causes may have greater public health relevance for universal prevention strategies (Knox et al., 2004).

Ecological studies, either using cross-national or cross-regional correlations or within-country time series analysis, allow examination of the relationship between regional or national aggregate data on elderly suicide rates and regional or national aggregate data on a range of parameters (e.g. socio-economic status) as potential risk or protective factors, and have major implications for public health. The findings of recent studies examining the relationship between elderly suicides and life expectancy, socio-economic status, income inequality, intelligence and educational attainment, fertility rates, urbanisation, societal crime,

[1] Address for correspondence: West London Mental Health NHS Trust, Uxbridge Road Southall Middlesex UB1 3EU United Kingdom; Telephone; 44 208 354 8140, Fax: 44 208 354 8898; E-mail: ajit.shah@wlmht.nhs.uk.

unemployment rates, gender inequality, population size, growth and dependency ratios, mental health service funding and provision and degree of human development are described.

Life-Expectancy

Increased child mortality rates and reduced the life expectancy were associated with elderly suicide rates in a recent cross-national ecological study (Shah et al., 2008a). Given that suicide rates generally increase with age (Shah and De, 1998; Shah, 2007a), increased child mortality and reduced life expectancy will result in fewer people reaching the age of increased risk for suicide. This is particularly likely in societies with low socio-economic status (Shah et al., 2008a; 2007b). This, in turn, will result in a reduced number of elderly suicides in countries with low socio-economic status. Also, selective survival of those at reduced risk of suicide in old age due to genetic or constitutional factors may further compound this trend (Suh and Shah, 2001). Moreover, in societies with low socio-economic status, those who do survive into old age may be at reduced risk of suicide because they may be able to better tolerate additional hardship in old age due to life-long exposure to adversity (Lindesay, 1991; Seiden, 1981), and this may also reduce the elderly suicide rate. This has been offered as an explanation for the low suicide rate among elderly African Americans and native Americans in the United States because they often have a life-long history of socio-economic deprivation (McIntosh, 1984). The significant positive correlations between suicide rates in both sexes in both the elderly age-bands and the proportion of elderly in the population also supports this hypothesis because increased life expectancy increases the proportion of elderly in the population (Shah et al., 2008a).

Socio-Economic Status and Income Inequality

Income inequality was associated with increased suicide rates in men over the age of 55 years in developed countries (Cutright and Fernquist, 2000), in both sexes in the general population in the United States (Kowalski et al., 1987), in both sexes up to the age of 75 years in Japan (Fukuda et al., 2005), and in both sexes over the age of 65 years in a cross-national study (Shah et al., 2008b). However, in England and Wales income inequality better correlated with suicide rates in younger men then in the elderly (Gunnell et al., 2003). Moreover, other markers of economic adversity were associated with increased suicide rates in males of all ages in Australia, although the opposite was observed for females (Berk et al., 2006). Also, some markers of economic adversity were differentially associated with suicide rates in different age-bands, including higher housing loan interest rates being associated with higher suicide rates in younger people but lower suicide rates in older people (Berk et al., 2006). Furthermore, suicide rates in females and older age groups were less influenced by indices of deprivation in England (Rezaeian et al., 2005). A study of 60 countries reported a positive correlation between gross national domestic product (GDP), a measure of socio-economic status, and suicide rates in both sexes in the general population (Zhang, 1998). However, in a study of 47 medium and high income countries, elderly suicide rates were negatively correlated with the GDP and were higher in countries with declining GDP (Kiemo,

2004). Furthermore, a decline in elderly suicide rates over time in England and Wales was associated with an increase in the GDP (Gunnell et al., 2003). Suicide rates in both sexes in the general population (Kennedy et al., 1999) and in the elderly (Whitley et al., 1999; Shah et al., 2002) were associated with socio-economic deprivation in England.

INTELLIGENCE AND EDUCATIONAL ATTAINMENT

General population suicide rates were positively correlated with intelligence levels in large cross-national studies (Lester, 2003; Voracek, 2004), and in individual countries including Belarus (Voracek, 2005a), United States (US) (Voracek, 2006a), Denmark (Voracek, 2006b) and Austria (Voracek, 2006c). However, this relationship was absent in other countries including France (Lester, 1993), Ireland (Lester, 1995), the United Kingdom (Lester, 1995) and Germany (Voracek, 2006d). A cross-national study of 48 Eurasian countries, the only study of elderly suicide rates, reported a positive correlation between elderly suicide rates and intelligence (Voracek, 2005b).

General population suicide rates in Japan (Otsu et al., 2005), Lithuania (Kalediene et al., 2006), and men in eight European countries (Lorant et al., 2005) were negatively correlated with educational attainment. Moreover, general population suicide rates in the US were observed to have no correlation (Saucer, 1993), positive correlation (Kowalski et al., 1987) and negative correlation (Abel and Kruger, 2005) with educational attainment; the latter observation may have been an artifact due to inter-state migration amongst the US adult population (Voracek, 2006e). Furthermore, general population suicide rates among African Americans (Lester 1990-1991) and in India (Mayer, 2003) positively correlated with educational attainment (Lester 1990-1991). A Canadian ecological study, the only study of elderly suicide rates, observed a negative correlation between educational attainment and suicide rates in elderly females (Agbayewa et al., 1998).

Voracek (2006f), based on data from cross-national studies, proposed that the relationship between intelligence and suicide rates in the general population and in the elderly followed an exponential-fit model rather than a linear-fit model. However, this exponential-fit model does not fully explain an absence of a relationship between suicide rates and intelligence in aggregate-level studies within several countries. Given the strong relationship between intelligence and educational attainment (Voracek, 2006a), this exponential-fit model also does not fully explain the observed relationships between suicide and both high and low levels of educational attainment in aggregate-level studies. One reason for this may be that aggregate-level studies have primarily used measures of linear correlation (Agbayewa et al., 1998). A Canadian ecological study, using measures of linear correlation, acknowledged that a possible non-linear relationship between elderly suicide rates and educational attainment may have been missed (Agbayewa et al., 1998). A recent cross-national study demonstarted a curvilinear (U-shaped) relationship between elderly suicide rates in both sexes and the Education Index, an aggregate measure of educational attianment, fitting a quadratic equation (Shah and Chaterjee, 2008).

Fertility Rates

Time series analysis observed negative correlations between birth rates and general population suicide rates in Canada (Leenaars et al., 1993, Leenaars and Lester, 1999; Bridges and Pearson, 2000), United States (Lester and Yang, 1992; Leenaars et al., 1993; Lester, 1994a), Germany (Wiedenmann and Weyerer, 1994), England and Wales (Lester, 1994b), Spain (Lester and Garcia, 1995), Finland (Lester, 1994c) and Denmark (Lester, 1994c; Lester, 1999); and, one cross-national study of 45 countries also reported similar findings (Stack, 1980). However, positive correlations between birth rates and general population suicide rates were observed in Puerto Rico (Lester, 1994b), Norway (Lester, 1994c) and Sweden (Lester, 1994c). Moreover, fertility rates were also negatively correlated with suicide rates in males and females under the age of 45 years (but not those over the age of 45 years), in the United States, over a 50-year period (Lester and Yang, 1992). The only study of elderly, a large cross-national study, observed a negative correlation between elderly suicide rates in both sexes and fertility rates (Shah, 2008a).

Urbanisation

A cross-national (Simpson and Conklin, 1989) and a single country (Stack, 1993) study reported a positive correlation between urbanisation and general population suicide rates. However, studies from advanced industrialised countries, including suicide rates in the general population in the United States (US) (Kowalski et al., 1987) and male suicide rates in the general population in Japan (Araki and Murata, 1986; Otsu et al., 2004), reported a negative correlation. Moreover, a large cross-national study reported no such relationship (Zhang, 1998). Stack (1982, 2000) explained these conflicting findings by proposing a curvilinear (quadratic) relationship, whereby the suicide rate would initially increase in the early stages of urbanisation due to social disruption following migration from rural to urban areas. Thereafter, the suicide rate would plateau, over several generations, as the new urban dwellers begin to adjust to living in urban areas (Stack, 1982, 2000). This adjustment may ultimately lead to a gradual reduction in the suicide rate (Stack, 1982, 2000). Stack (2000) argued that this curvilinear relationship was supported by a longitudinal study of general population suicide rates in Finland (Stack, 1993). A recent cross-national study demonstrated a curvilinear (inverted U-shaped curve) relationship between male suicide rates in both the elderly age-bands and the percentage of the population living in urban areas fitting a quadratic equation (Shah, 2008b); a similar curvilinear relationship was observed for elderly females, but the relationships was not statistically significant.

Societal Crime

The only study, a cross-national study, on elderly suicide rates and aggregate national crime rates, reported negative correlations between elderly suicide rates and the percentage of the population victimised by the crime of robbery and property crime (Shah, 2008c).

UNEMPLOYMENT

Within-country ecological studies of geographical areas or time-series aggregate-level studies from Japan (Yamasaki et al., 2005), Trinidad (Hutchinson and Simeon, 1997), Ireland (Daly et al., 1996), Northern Ireland (Snyder, 1992), Canada (Leenaars et al., 1993), United States (Lester and Yang, 1992; Lester, 1994d), United Kingdom (Pritchard, 1992) and some European Community countries (Pritchard, 1992) have reported an association between unemployment and higher general population suicide rates, particularly in men in the younger age groups. The Japanese study reported an unemployment and lower suicide rates in elderly women (Yamasaki et al., 2005). However, a recent large cross-national study observed an absence of any relationship between elderly suicide rates and societal unemployment rates (Shah, 2008d).

GENDER INEQUALITY

Two proxy measures of gender equality (the gender empowerment measure value and the gender-related development index – both national-level aggregate measures developed by the United Nations) did not account for significant variation in the male to female sex ratio of elderly suicide rates in a recent large cross-national study (Shah, 2008e).

POPULATION SIZE, GROWTH AND DEPENDENCY RATIOS

A positive correlations between elderly suicide rates and elderly population size and the proportion of elderly in the population has been reported in recent cross-national studies (Kiemo, 2004; Shah et al., 2008a).

The only study, a cross-national study, examining the relationship between elderly suicide rates and national aggregate-level elderly dependency ratios (the ratio of those over the age of 65 years to those under the age of 65 years), reported a positive correlation (Shah et al., 2008b).

The only study, a cross-national study, examining the relationship between elderly suicide rates and average annual national population growth observed a curvilinear (U-shaped curve) relationship fitting a quadratic equation (Shah, 2008f).

MENTAL HEALTH FUNDING AND SERVICE PROVISION

In a recent cross-national study there was no relationship between elderly suicide rates and different measures of mental health policy, except they were increased in countries with a substance abuse policy (Shah and Bhat, 2008a). The same study reported that elderly suicide rates were higher in countries with greater provision of mental health services, including the number of psychiatric beds, psychiatrists and psychiatric nurses, and the availability of training in mental health for primary care professionals (Shah and Bhat, 2008a). A re-analysis of the same data set observed that the relationship between the elderly suicide rates and the percentage of the total health budget spent on mental health, the total number of psychiatric beds per 10,000 population and the total number of psychiatrists per 10,000 population were curvilinear (inverted U-shaped curve) and fitted a quadratic equation (Shah and Bhat, 2008b). A decline in elderly suicide rates in England and Wales was associated with measures of improved healthcare for the elderly (Gunnell et al., 2003; Lodhi and Shah, 2005) including an increase in the number of general practitioners, hospital medical staff, out-patient appointments for mental illness, and field social workers and day centre staff (Lodhi and Shah, 2005). Additionally, a decline in elderly suicide rates in England and Wales was associated with an increase in prescription rates of antidepressants (Gunnell et al., 2003; Lodhi and Shah, 2004), including selective serotonin reuptake inhibitors (Lodhi and Shah, 2004).

Human Development Index

The Human Development Index (HDI), developed by the United Nations, is a composite index measuring the average achievements in a given country on three basic dimensions of human development: a long and healthy life, as measured by life expectancy; educational attainment, as measured by the adult literacy rate and the combined gross enrollment ratio for primary, secondary and tertiary schools; and, a decent standard of living, as measured by the GDP. Moreover, the UN ranks countries by the degree of development measured by the HDI. The only study, a recent cross-national study, examining the relationship between elderly suicide rates and HDI reported a curvilinear (inverted U-shaped curve) relationship fitting the quadratic equation (Shah, 2008f).

A Way Forward

Cross-national data on suicide rates should be viewed with caution because: data are not available from all countries (Moscicki, 1995; Wasserman et al., 2005); the validity of this data is unclear (Diekstra, 1989; Wasserman et al., 2005); the legal criteria for the proof of suicide vary between countries and in different regions within a country (Shah and Ganesvaran, 1994; Wasserman et al., 2005); some countries, particularly low-income countries, may have poor death registration facilities (Shah and Ganesvaran, 1994); and, cultural and religious factors and stigma attached to suicide in some countries may lead to under-reporting of suicides (Wasserman et al., 2005; Abrahams et al., 2005). Another limitation of utilising national aggregate data is the possibility of missing variations in suicide rates in different regions within a country (Rehkopf and Buka, 2006). Data on socio-economic status and health-related measures should also be viewed with caution because: the validity of this data is unclear; some countries may have poor registration facilities for data on health-related measures; some countries may have poor infrastructure for providing accurate financial data; and, their influence on social distribution of risk factors may be complex (Lynch et al., 2004). These latter concerns are more likely to be observed in low-income countries (Shah et al., 2008a).

Caution should be exercised in the attribution of a causal relationship and the direction of this relationship because of the cross-sectional and ecological study design whereby the findings are subject to ecological fallacy. Nevertheless, they allow generation of potentially testable aetiological hypotheses. One example pertaining to the findings of a recent cross-national ecological study were used to develop a potentially testable theoretical and hypothetical four sequential stage model to explain the curvilinear relationship between elderly suicide rates and the HDI. Similar models have been proposed to explain the relationship between socio-economic status and cross-national variations in the prevalence of dementia (Suh and Shah, 2001) and other mental disorders in old age (Shah, 2007b). An empirical assumption, whereby each country progresses through each of the four proposed developmental stages during it's development, was made. The model assumed that both elderly suicide rates and the HDI of countries can be dichotomised into two groups: high and low.

1. Low Elderly Suicide Rate-Low Human Development Society Stage

There is consistent evidence of an association between low elderly suicide rates and poor socio-economic status and greater income inequality from cross-national (Zhang, 1998; Simpson and Conklin, 1989; Shah *et al.,* 2008a) and within-country (Kowlaski *et al.,* 1987) studies. Societies with low socio-economic status and greater income inequality have poorly developed healthcare services (Shah *et al.,* 2008a; Shah, 2007b). Poorly developed healthcare services may mediate an increase in child mortality rates as observed by negative correlations between markers of development of healthcare services and child mortality rates (Suh and Shah, 2001; Shah *et al.,* 2008a; Shah, 2007b). Child mortality rates were also negatively correlated with the GDP and positively correlated with the Gini coefficient, a measure of income inequality (Zhang, 1998; Shah *et al.,* 2008a; Shah, 2007b). Increased child mortality rates will, in turn, reduce the life expectancy (Zhang, 1998; Shah *et al.,* 2008a; Shah, 2007b). Given that suicide rates generally increase with age (Shah and De, 1998; Shah, 2007a), reduced life expectancy will result in fewer people reaching the age of increased risk for suicide in countries with low socio-economic status, and result in a reduced number of elderly suicides in such countries. This is supported by positive correlations between life expectancy and suicide rates in the elderly (Shah *et al.,* 2008a) and the general population (Zhang, 1998) in cross-national studies. Moreover, in societies with low socio-economic status, the elderly may be at reduced risk of suicide because they may have greater tolerance of additional hardship in old age due to life-long exposure to adversity (Lindesay, 1991; Seiden, 1981); this has been suggested as an explanation for low elderly suicide rates among African Americans and native Americans in the US (McIntosh, 1984). The positive correlation between elderly suicide rates and the proportion of elderly in the population (Keimo, 2004; Shah *et al.,* 2008a,b) further supports this hypothesis because increased life expectancy increases the proportion of elderly in the population. Furthermore, correlations between life expectancy and GDP (positive) and Gini coefficient (negative) have also been reported (Zhang, 1998; Keimo, 2004; Shah *et al.,* 2008a; Shah, 2007b).

The above approach is consistent with a previously developed model with five sequential stages (Shah *et al.,* 2008a): (i) presence of a low socio-economic status; (ii) low socio-economic status leading to poorly developed healthcare services; (iii) poorly developed healthcare services may interact, mediate and modify other factors and contribute to increased child mortality rates; (iv) increased child mortality rates leading to reduced life expectancy; and, (v) reduced life expectancy leading to fewer people reaching the age of increased risk of suicide, and resulting in low elderly suicide rates in societies with low socio-economic status.

2. High Elderly Suicide Rate-Low Human Development Society Stage

Improvement in the development of healthcare services are associated with improvement in the socio-economic status of countries (Shah *et al.,* 2008a; Shah, 2007b). Improved healthcare services were observed to reduce child mortality (Shah *et al.,* 2008a; Shah, 2007b). Reduction in child mortality rates will, in turn, increase the life expectancy (Zhang, 1998; Shah *et al*., 2008a). This, in turn, will result in greater number of subjects reaching the age of increased risk of suicide and an increase in elderly suicide rates. This is supported by positive correlations between life expectancy and suicide rates in the elderly (Shah *et al.,* 2008a) and general population (Zhang, 1998). This approach is also consistent with the five stage sequential model described above in the section on Low elderly suicide rates – low human development society stage (Shah *et al.,* 2008a). This will lead to a gradual transition from low elderly suicide rate-low human development society stage to a high elderly suicide rate-low human development society stage.

3. High Elderly Suicide Rate-High Human Development Society Stage

As societies develop, a change from lower to higher human development status will occur. This will lead to further improvements in the development of healthcare services as observed by positive correlations between GDP and markers of development of healthcare, and negative correlations between the Gini coefficent and these variables (Shah *et al.,* 2008a; Shah, 2007b). Further improvement in healthcare services has been observed to facilitate further reductions in child mortality rates (Zhang, 1998; Shah *et al.,* 2008a; Shah, 2007b). Further reductions in child mortality rates will, in turn, further increase the life expectancy (Zhang, 1998; Shah *et al.,* 2008a; Shah, 2007b). This, in turn, will result in increasing number of subjects reaching the age of increased risk of suicide; the positive correlations between life expectancy and suicide rates in the elderly (Shah *et al.,* 2008a) and general population (Zhang, 1998) further supports this. Moreover, the protective effects of life-long adversity on elderly suicide rates (Seiden, 1981; Lindesay, 1991; McIntosh, 1984) is likely to be less prevalent in countries with higher socio-economic status. The composite effect of these changes will increase the number of individuals at increased risk of suicide in old age in socio-economically more developed countries. This approach is also consistent with the five stage sequential model described above in the section on Low elderly suicide rates – low human development society stage (Shah *et al.,* 2008a). This will lead to a gradual transition from the high elderly suicide rate-low human development society stage to a high elderly suicide rate-high human development society stage.

4. Low Elderly Suicide Rate-High Human Development Society Stage

Theoretically, in socio-economically well developed countries, due to further reduction in child mortality rates and increase in life expectancy, greater number of people would reach the age of increased of suicide, and consequently lead to higher elderly suicide rates. However, in socio-economically well developed countries, including Italy, Netherlands, Norway, United Kingdom and United States, elderly suicide rates are comparatively low (Shah *et al.,* 2007) and have declined over time (Shah *et al.,* 2008c). The five stage sequential model described above in the section on Low elderly suicide rates – low human development society stage (Shah *et al.,* 2008a) appears not apply to socio-economically well developed countries. In socio-economically well developed countries, elderly suicide rates may progressively decline over many years due to improved efforts to control the risk factors for elderly suicides, enhance protective factors for elderly suicides, and advances in medical care. Ultimately, this will lead to a gradual transition from a high elderly suicide rate-high human development society stage to a low elderly suicide rate-high human development society stage.

England and Wales could be considered to be at this developmental stage. In England and Wales, elderly suicide rates were higher in areas with high socio-economic deprivation (Whitley *et al.,* 1999; Shah *et al.,* 2002) and high social fragmentation (Whitley *et al.,* 1999). A decline in elderly suicide rates over time in England and Wales was associated with an increase in GDP (Gunnell *et al.,* 2003). Therefore, in socio-economically well developed societies further improvement in socio-economic status appears to be an important factor in reducing elderly suicide rates. What is the mechanism for the reduction in elderly suicide rates due to improved socio-economic status?

Almost all elderly suicide victims have mental illness, and up to 90% have depression (Shah and De, 1998). A significant number of elderly suicide victims in socio-economically well developed countries consult their general practitioner or psychiatrist or contact mental health services between one week and six months prior to the suicide (Conwell *et al.,* 1991; Catell and Jolley, 1995; Vassilas and Morgan, 1993, 1994). This offers opportunity for identification and treatment of the mental illness. Thus, the availability of appropriate healthcare services may be an important factor contributing to elderly suicide rates. High suicide rates in rural China and Hong Kong, in part, have been attributed to lack of mental health services and poorly developed social welfare and benefit systems (Yip and Tan, 1998; Jianlin, 2000; Yip, 2001; Yip *et al.,* 2000). Socio-economically well developed societies generally have well developed healthcare services, and this is supported by the observed positive correlations between GDP and markers development of healthcare and negative correlations between the Gini coefficent and these variables (Shah *et al.,* 2008a; Shah, 2007b). Decline in elderly suicide rates in England and Wales was associated with measures of improved healthcare for the elderly (Gunnell *et al.,* 2003; Lodhi and Shah, 2005) including an increase in the number of general practitioners, hospital medical staff, out-patient appointments for mental illness, field social workers and day centre staff (Lodhi and Shah, 2005). Reduction in elderly suicide rates in Singapore and urban China have been attributed to improved healthcare and welfare services for the elderly (Kua *et al.,* 2003; Yip *et al.,* 2005). Socio-economically well developed countries are also more likely to have appropriate healthcare facilities to promptly resusitate those who have attempted suicides, thus further reducing elderly suicide rates. Physical illness is an important risk factor for elderly suicides

(Catell, 1988; Catell and Jolley, 1995), and socio-economically well developed societies generally have appropriate healthcare care facilities for the treatment of physical illness, thus helping to further reduce elderly suicide rates.

Some recent public health initiatives in the United Kingdom may be responsible for the improvement in the health structure by improving detection and treatment of individuals at risk of suicide. Such initiatives included legislation encouraging general practitioners to offer annual physical and mental examination to those over the age of 75 years, the Defeat Depression Campaign organised by the Royal College of Psychiatrist and the Royal College of General Practitioners, the governmental "Our Healthier Nation" suicide reduction targets, the National Confidential Enquiry into Suicides and Homicides, the National Service Frameworks for Mental Health and for Older People, and the National Suicide Prevention Strategy (Hoxey and Shah, 2000; Shah *et al.,* 2001; Shah, 2007c). Additionally, a decline in elderly suicide rates in England and Wales was associated with an increase in prescription rates of antidepressants (Gunnell *et al.,* 2003; Lodhi and Shah, 2004), particularly selective serotonin reuptake inhibitors (Lodhi and Shah, 2004); this has also been observed in Sweden (Carlsten *et al.,* 1999) and Australia (Hall *et al.,* 2003). This change may have been a direct result of the various initiatives described above, which may have promoted health-seeking behaviour among patients at risk of suicide and improved prescribing patterns for antidepressants amongst doctors. Furthermore, such public health initiatives are more likely to be instigated in countries at a more advanced stage of socio-economic development because they require substantive funding.

REFERENCES

Abrahams VJ, Abrahams S, Jacob KS (2005) Suicide in the elderly in Kanyambadi block, Tamil Nadu, South India. *International Journal of Geriatric Psychiatry*, 20, 953-955.

Abel EL, Kruger ML (2005) Educational attainment and suicide rates in the United States. *Psychological Reports*, 97, 25-28.

Agbayewa OM, Marion SA, Wiggins S (1998) Socioeconomic factors associated with suicide in elderly populations in British Columbia: an 11-year review. *Canadian Journal of Psychiatry,* 43, 829-836.

Araki S, Murata K. (1986) Social life factors affecting suicide in Japanese men and women. Suicide and Life Threatening Behaviour, 16, 458-468.

Berk M, Dodd S, Henry M (2006) The effect of macroeconomic variables on suicide. *Psychological Medicine,* 36, 181-189.

Bridges FS, Perason LC. (2004) Use of the same and a longer time series to replicate David Lester's study of suicide and birth rates in Canada. *Perceptual Motor Skill,* 98, 1090-1091.

Carlsten A, Waern M, Allebeck P. (1999). Suicides by drug poisoning among the elderly in Sweden 1969-1996. *Social Psychiatry and Psychiatric Epidemiology*, 34, 609-614.

Cattell H, Jolley D (1995) One hundred cases of suicide in the elderly. *British Journal of Psychiatry*, 166, 451-457.

Conwell Y, Olsen K, Caine ED, Flannery C (1991) Suicide in later life: psychological autopsy findings. *International Psychogeriatrics*, 3, 59-66.

Cutright P, Fernquist RM (2000) Effects of social integration, period, region, and culture of suicide on male age-specific suicide rates: 20 developed countries, 1955-1898. *Social Science Research*, 29, 148-172.

Daly C, Kelleher MJ, Crowley MJ, Daly M, Keohane B, Daly F, McLeavey BC. (1996) Suicide levels in Cork City 1987/1991. *Irish Medical Journal*, 89, 99-101.

Diekstra RFW (1989) Suicide and attemptede suicide: an international perspective. *Acta Psychiatrica Scandinavica,* 80 (Suppl 354), 1-24.

Fukuda Y, Nakamura K, Takano T (2005) Cause-specific mortality differences across socioeconomic position of municipalities in Japan, 1973-1977 and 1993-1998: increased importance of injury and suicide in inequality for ages under 75. *International Journal of Epidemiology*, 34, 100-109.

Gunnell D, Middleston N, Whitley E, Dorling D, Frankel S (2003) Why are suicide rates rising in young men but falling in the elderly? – a time-series analysis of trends in England and Wales 1950-1998. *Social Science and Medicine,* 57, 595-611.

Hall W, Mant A, Mitchell P, Rendle VA, Hickie IB, McManus P. (2003). Association between antidepressant prescribing and suicide in Australia, 1991-2000: trend analysis. *British Medical Journal*, 326, 1008-1011.

Harwood D, Hawton K, Hope T, Jacoby R (2001) Psychiatric disorder and personality factors associated with suicide in older people: a descriptive and case-control study. International *Journal of Geriatric Psychiatry*, 16, 155-165.

Hoxey K, Shah AK. (2000). Recent trends in suicide rates and methods in England and Wales. *International Journal of Geriatric Psychiatry*, 15, 274-279.

Jianlin J. (2000). Suicide rates and mental health services in modern China. Crisis, 21, 118-121.

Kalediene R, Starkuviene S, Petrauskiene J (2006) Social dimension of mortality from external causes in Lithuania: do education and place of residence matter. Soz Praventivmed, 51, 232-239.

Kiemo K (2004) Towards a socio-economic and demographic theory of elderly suicides: a comparison of 49 countries at various stages of development. www.soc.ou.se/publications/fulltext/diss2003-3.pdf. Viewed 2 Febraury 2007.

Kennedy HG, Iveson RC, Hill O (1999) Violence, homicide and suicide: strong correlation and wide variation across districts. *British Journal of Psychiatry*, 175, 462-466.

Knox KL, Conwell Y, Caine ED (2004) If suicide is a public health problem, what are we doing to prevent it? *American Journal of Public Health*, 94, 37-45.

Kowalski GS, Faupel CE, Starr PD (1987) Urbanisation and suicides: a study of American Counties. Social Forces, 66, 85-101.

Kua EH, Ko SM, Ng TP. (2003). Recent trends in elderly suicide rates in a multi-ethnic Asian city. *International Journal of Geriatric Psychiatry,* 18, 533-536.

Leenaars AA, Lester D. (1999) Domestic integration and suicide in the provinces of Canada. *Crisis,* 20, 59-63.

Leenaars AA, Yang B, Lester D. (1993) The effect of domestic and economic stress on suicide rates in Canada and the United States. *Journal of Clinical Psychology,* 49, 918-921.

Lester D (1990-1991) Mortality from suicide and homocide for African Americans in the USA: A regional analysis. Omega: *Journal of Death and Dying*, 22, 216-226.

Lester D (1993) Intelligence and suicide in France: an ecological study. *Psychological Reports*, 73, 1226.

Lester D. (1994a) Social integration and suicide in Puerto Rico and the United States. PRHSJ, 13, 39.

Lester D. (1994b) Comparing the changing suicide rate in Singapore with the rates in England/Wales and the USA, 1950-1985. *Singapore Medical Journal,* 35, 490-491.

Lester D. (1994c) The variation of suicide rates over time in Scandinavia. *Scandinavian Journal of Social Medicine*, 22, 160-161.

Lester D. (1994d) Suicide and unemployment: a monthly analysis. *Psychological Reports*, 75, 602.

Lester D (1995) Intelligence and suicide in Ireland and the United Kingdom. *Psychological Reports,* 77, 122.

Lester D. (1999) Correlates of suicide rates calculated in different ways: Denmark 1950-1985. *Perceptual Motor Skills*, 89, 172.

Lester D (2003) National estimates of IQ and suicide and homocide rates. *Perceptual and Motor Skills*, 97, 206.

Lester D, Garcia JMG (1995) Suicide and domestic integration in Spain: the effect of the source of suicide statistics. *Psychological Reports,* 77, 1218.

Lester D, Yang B. (1992) Fertility and suicide rates: a time series analysis in the United States. *Journal of Biosocial Science*, 24, 97-101.

Lindesay J (1991) Suicide in the elderly. *International Journal of Geriatric Psychiatry,* 6, 355-361.

Lorant V (2005) Socio-economic inequalities in suicide: a European comparative study. *British Journal of Psychiatry,* 187, 49-54.

Lodhi L, Shah AK. Psychotropic prescriptions and elderly suicide rates. *Medicine, Science and the Law*. 2004; 44: 236-244.

Lodhi L, Shah AK. (2005) Factors associated with the recent decline in suicide rates in England and Wales. 1985-1998. *Medicne, Science and the Law*, 45, 115-120.

Lynch J, Davey Smith G, Harpe S et al (2004) Is income inequality a determinant of population health? Part 1. A systematic review. Millbank Q, 82, 5-99.

Mayer P (2003) Female equality and suicide in the Indian states. *Psychological Reports*, 92, 1022-1028.

McIntosh JL (1984) Components of the decline in elderly suicides: suicide in young old and old old by race and sex. *Death Education*, 8, 113-124.

Moscicki EK (1995) North American perspectives: epidemiology of suicide. *International Psychogeriatrics*, 7, 137-148.

Otsu A, Araki S, Sakai R, Yokoyama K, Voorhees AS (2004) Effects of urbanization, economic development, and migration of workers on suicide mortality in Japan. *Social Sciences and Medicine*, 58, 1137-1146.

Rehkopf DH, Buka SL (2006) The association between suicide and the socio-economic characteristics of geographical areas: a systematic review. *Psychological Medicine,* 36, 145-157.

Rezaeian M, Dunn G, St Leger S, Appleby L (2005) The ecological association between suicide rates and indices of deprivation in English local authorities. *Social Psychiatry and Psychiatric Epidemiology,* 40, 785-791,

Saucer PR (1993) Education and suicide: the quality of life among modern Americans. *Psychological Reports*, 73, 637-638.

Seiden RH (1981) Mellowing with age: factors affecting the non-white suicide rate. *International Journal of Ageing and Human Development*, 13, 265-284.

Shah AK (2007a) The relationship between suicide rates and age: an analysis of multinational data from the World Health Organisation. *International Psychogeriatrics*, 19. 1141-1152.

Shah AK (2007b) The importance of socio-economic status of countries for mental disorders in old age: a development of an epidemiological transition model. *International Psychogeriatrics*, 19, 785-787.

Shah AK (2007c). Elderly suicide rates in the United Kingdom: trends from 1979 to 2002. *Medicine, Science and the Law*, 47, 56-60.

Shah AK. (2008a) Association of suicide rates in elderly persons with fertility rates. *Psychological Reports*, 102, 369-376.

Shah AK (2008b). A cross-national study of the relationship between elderly suicide rates and urbanization. *Suicide and Life Threatening Behaviour*. In Press.

Shah AK (2008c). Possible realtion between suicide rates of elderly with societal crime: a cross-national study. *Psychological Reports*, 102, 95-98.

Shah AK. (2008d) Possible relation of elderly suicide rates with unemployment in society: a cross-national study. *Psychological Reports,* 102, 398-400.

Shah AK. (2008e) Association of suicide rates for elderly age bands with gender equality. *Psychological Reports*, 102, 887-892.

Shah AK. (2008e) The relationship between population growth and elderly suicide rates. A cross-national study. *International Psychogeriatrics*. In Press.

Shah AK (2008f). The relationship between elderly suicide rates and the Human Development Index: a cross-national study of secondary data from the WHO and the United Nations. *International Psychogeriatrics*. In press.

Shah AK, Bhat R. (2008a)The relationship between elderly suicide rates and mental health funding, service provision and national policy: a cross-national study. *International Psychogeriatrics*, 20, 605-615.

Shah AK, Bhat R. (2008b) Are elderly suicide rates improved by increased provision of mental health service resources? *International Psychogeriatrics*, 20, 1230-1237.

Shah AK, Bhat R, MacKenzie S, Koen C. (2007). Elderly suicide rates: cross-national comparisons and association with sex and elderly age-bands. *Medicine, Science and the Law*, 47, 244-252.

Shah AK, Bhat R, MacKenzie S, Koen C. (2008a) A cross-national study of the relationship between elderly suicide rates and life expectancy and markers of socio-economic status and healthcare status. *International Psychogeriatrics,* 20, 347-360.

Shah AK, Bhat R, MacKenzie S, Koen C. (200*c). Elderly suicide rates: cross-national comparisons over a ten year time period. *International Psychogeriatrics*. In Press.

Shah AK, Chaterjee S. (2008) Is there a relationship between elderly suicide rates and educational attainment? A cross-national study. Ageing and Mental Health. In Press.

Shah AK, De T (1998) Suicide and the elderly. *International Journal of Psychiatry in Clinical Practice*, 2, 3-17.

Shah AK, Ellanchanny N, Collinge T. (2001). Trends in age band-specific suicide rates in the elderly. *Medicine, Science and the Law*, 41, 102-106.

Shah AK, Ganesvaran T (1994) Suicide in the elderly. In: Functional Psychiatric Disorders of the Elderly (Eds. Chiu E, Ames D). Cambridge, Cambridge University Press. Pgs 221-244.

Shah AK, MacKenzie S (2007) Disorders of ageing across cultures. In: Textbook of Cultural Psychiatry (Eds. Bhugra D and Bhui K). Cambridge, Cambridge University Press. Pgs 323-344.

Shah AK, Padayatchi M, Das K. (2008b) The relationship between elderly suicide rates and elderly dependency ratios: a cross-national study using data from the WHO data bank. *International Psychogeriatrics*, 20, 594-604.

Shah R, Uren Z, Baker A, Majeed A (2002) Trends in suicide from drug overdose in the elderly in England and Wales, 1993-1999. *International Journal of Geriatric Psychiatry,* 17, 416-421.

Simpson M, Concklin G. (1989) Socio-economic development, suicide and religion: a test of Durkhiem's theory of religion and suicide. *Social Forces,* 67, 945-964.

Stack S (1980) Domestic integration and the rate of suicide: a comparative study. *Journal of Comparative Family Studies,* 11, 249-260.

Stack S. (1982) Suicide: a decade review of sociological literature. *Deviant Behaviour,* 4, 41-66.

Stack S. (1993) The effect of modernization on suicide in Finland, 1800-1985. *Sociological Perspective,* 36, 137-148.

Stack S. (2000) Suicide: a 15-year review of the sociological literature Part II: modernization and social integration perspectives. *Suicide and Life Threatening Behaviour*, 30, 163-176.

Suh GH, Shah AK (2001) A review of the epidemiological transition in dementia – cross-national comparisons of the indices related to Alzheimer's disease and vascular dementia. *Acta Psychiatrica Scandinavica*, 104, 4-11.

Synder ML. (1992) Unemployment and suicide rate in Northern Ireland. *Psychological Reports,* 70, 1116-1118.

Vassilas CA, Morgan HG. (1993).General practitioner's contact with victims of suicide. *British Medical Journal*, 307, 300-301.

Vassilas CA, Morgan HG. (1994) Elderly suicides' contact with their general practitioner before death. *International Journal of Geriatric Psychiatry*, 9, 1008-1009.

Voracek M (2004) National intelligence and suicide rate: an ecological study of 85 countries. *Personality and Individual Differences,* 37, 543-553.

Voracek M (2005a) The social ecology of Intelligence and suicide in Belarus. *Journal of Social Psychology*, 145, 613-617.

Voracek M (2005b) National intelligence, suicide rate in the elderly, and a threshold intelligence for suicidality: an ecological study of 48 Eurasian countries. *Journal of Biosocial Science*, 37, 721-740.

Voracek M (2006a) Social ecology of intelligence and suicide in the United States. *Perceptual and Motor Skills*, 102, 767-775.

Voracek M (2006b) Regional intelligence and suicide rate in Denmark. *Psychological Reports*, 98, 671-674.

Voracek M (2006c) Smart or suicidal? The social ecology of intelligence and suicide in Austria. *Death Studies,* 30, 471-485.

Voracek M (2006d) Regional intelligence and suicide rate in Germany. *Perceptual and Motor Skills*, 103, 2, 639-642.

Voracek M (2006e) Educational attainment, intelligence, interstate migration, and suicide rates in the United States: rejoinder to Abel and Kruger. *Psychological Reports,* 98, 608-610.

Voracek M (2006f) Exponential fitting of suicide rate and national intelligence estimates. *Perceptual and Motor Skills*, 102, 896-898.

Wasserman D, Cheng Q, Jiang GX (2005) Global suicide rates among young people aged 15-19. World Psychiatry, 4, 114-120.

Whitley E, Gunnell D, Dorling D, Smith GD (1999) Ecological study of social fragmentation, poverty, and suicide. *British Medical Journal*, 319, 1034-1037.

Yamasaki A, Sakai R, Shirakawa T. (2005) Low income, unemployment, and suicide mortality rates for middle-age persons in Japan. *Psychological Reports*, 96, 337-248.

Yip PSF. (2001). An epidemiological profile of suicides in Beijing, Chine. Suicide and Life-*Threatening Behaviour*, 31, 62-70.

Yip PSF, Callanan C, Yuen HP (2000). Urban/rural and gender differences in suicide rates: East and West. *Journal of Affective Disorders*, 57, 99-106.

Yip PSF, Liu KY, Hu J. Song XM (2005). Suicide rates in China during a decade of rapid social change. *Social Psychiatry and Psychiatric Epidemiology*, 40, 792-798.

Yip PSF, Tan RCE (1998). Suicides in Hong Kong and Singapore: a tale of two cities. *International Journal of Social Psychiatry*, 44, 267-279.

Zhang J (1998) Suicide in the world: toward a population increase theory of suicide. *Death Studies*, 22, 525-539.

In: Psychiatric Research Trends: Dreams and Geriatric Psychiatry ISBN 978-1-60741-760-6
Editors: Daniella M. Montez, pp.133-144

Chapter 8

DREAMING DURING ANESTHESIA

M. J. Paech[1] and K. Leslie[2]

[1]Professor of Obstetric Anaesthesia, The School of Medicine and Pharmacology, The University of Western Australia, Perth, Western Australia, Australia

[2]Head of Research, Department of Anaesthesia and Pain Management, Royal Melbourne Hospital and Professorial Fellow, Department of Pharmacology, University of Melbourne, Melbourne, Victoria, Australia

ABSTRACT

Excluding awareness, which is the post-anesthesia recall of real events, dreaming during anesthesia can be defined as any recalled experience that occurred between induction of general anesthesia and the first return of consciousness after anesthesia. It is a common phenomenon (5-50%) that varies in incidence with the timing of the post-anesthesia interview. Dreaming is most frequently reported by women who are young, healthy, have home dream recall after sleep, receive short propofol-based anesthesia and who emerge from anesthesia rapidly.

Most dreams are short and neutral or pleasant in content, the latter being related to work, family and recreational activities. Rarely, the dream content suggests a 'near-miss' awareness experience that resulted from an inadequate depth of anesthesia and transient return of consciousness, but most dreams appear to occur during a sleep state in the period just before initial arousal from unconsciousness at the end of anesthesia.

This chapter reviews the incidence of dreaming, factors influencing dreaming, the nature and content of dreams and their psychological impact, the timing of dreaming and the evidence as to whether it occurs during or after anesthesia. To date, research about dreaming during anesthesia has largely involved observational clinical studies, but future neurophysiological research should provide more detailed understanding of what appears to be a common, not unpleasant and harmless event.

INTRODUCTION

Memory and Awareness During Anesthesia

General anesthetic drugs are a diverse group of chemicals that share the ability to suppress central nervous system (CNS) function. Aims of general anesthesia include rendering the patient immobile, less responsive to noxious (surgical) stimuli and in a state of reversible unconsciousness. The depth of the unconscious state varies throughout general anesthesia and it is now possible to incorporate the monitoring of cortical electroencephalographic (EEG) function (or more experimentally auditory-evoked responses or other measures) with clinical monitoring as a means of assessing the depth of anesthesia and reducing the risk of a return of consciousness during anesthesia [1,2]. The latter event may be associated with postoperative patient recall of actual intraoperative events, which is termed "awareness".

Although phrases pertaining to sleep are often used by anesthesiologists when referring to anesthesia ("You are going off to sleep now" or "See you when you wake up"), the patient cannot be woken from general anesthesia, because CNS activity is suppressed. In contrast, during sleep patients can be roused and the brain may be activated, especially during rapid-eye movement (REM) sleep. This is a period of vivid sensory dreaming, whereas dreams during non-REM sleep tend not to be hallucinatory or perceptual and are more likely to be ruminations on the past or future [3]. Common to states of sleep, drug-induced sedation and anesthesia is that memory function is impaired but memories can be formed [4-6].

During adequate anesthesia (an aim of which is amnesia for the intraoperative period) only the most basic memory function of implicit memory (memories of which we are unaware and which reveal themselves through changes in behaviour) is retained [6]. This function is termed perceptual priming (the temporarily increased activation of a word or idea in memory). Conceptual priming (the activation of related knowledge) is a more advanced function that requires conscious encoding of the stimulus and thus it does not persist at adequate depths of anesthesia. However, during very 'light' anesthesia consciousness may return and at low levels of stimulation approximately one-third of such patients who regain consciousness subsequently show explicit memory formation and thus experience "awareness" [5]. The incidence of awareness is influenced by a number of patient and anesthetic factors but occurs in approximately 1-2 per 1000 (0.1-0.2%) surgical patients [7]. In contrast, the incidence of dreaming during anesthesia is much higher, being reported by 3-50% of patients (both adults and children greater than 3 years of age) [2,6-12]. Although there is an association between awareness and dreaming, with patients who report dreaming also being more likely to experience awareness and those who have awareness also often reporting dreaming [12], the nature of the association is unclear. Indeed dreams during anesthesia very infrequently appear representative of 'near-miss' awareness or predecessors of explicit recall.

A Historical Perspective

Dreaming associated with anesthesia has been described since the inception of anesthesia almost 150 years ago [13]. Not surprisingly, historically dreaming has been considered to be 'near-miss' awareness, because until 25 years ago very light anesthesia, omitting either volatile inhaled or infused intravenous anesthetic drugs, was commonly used. The frequency of both dreaming and awareness was then much higher than now. Some of the first studies to systematically investigate dreaming during anesthesia found no cases of awareness but a 44-57% incidence of dreaming [14,15]. However, a reduction in incidence to 23% was observed when pre-anesthetic opioid was administered and to 0% when volatile anesthetic drugs were added [15].

Current anesthetic techniques include the administration of inhaled volatile or intravenous anesthetic drugs post-induction, to maintain anesthesia, and with these approaches the reported incidence is less, varying primarily with specific drug combinations, the characteristics of the patient population and assessment methods. In the past decade, the introduction of depth of anesthesia monitoring, particularly devices that apply proprietary algorithms based on population-based EEG data from anesthetized patients, has lead to an improvement in the ability of anesthesiologist to estimate the depth of anesthesia. Recently these tools have been used to investigate the timing of dreaming, in particular the relationship between dreaming and both the depth of anesthesia and the post-arousal state.

Many patients who remain conscious under regional anesthesia are also sedated. The sedative drugs used also cause dreaming of similar nature to dreams during general anesthesia [16] and unpleasant experiences also appear rare [17].

The content of dreams aroused interest soon after the introduction of anesthesia at the first demonstration of ether anesthesia in Boston, Massachusetts on October 16, 1846. This was no doubt largely because of anecdotal descriptions of amorous behaviour, sexual ideation and erotic dreams, especially among younger adult women [13]. The use of obscene language by women receiving chloroform caused a stir in 1849 and was well recognized by the 1850s [13]. These phenomena resurfaced after the introduction of the intravenous anesthetic drug propofol during the 1980s [18,19], although they are not exclusive to anesthetic drugs because sedative drugs such as the benzodiazepines and nitrous oxide have also been implicated.

CURRENT KNOWLEDGE

Predictors of Dreaming During Anesthesia

A number of factors influence the incidence and nature of dreaming, in particular the timing of questioning, the type of surgery, the method and depth of anesthesia, and the patient characteristics.

Dreams are easily forgotten. The recall of dreams falls over time during recovery from anesthesia, such that the incidence is higher at awakening from anesthesia than subsequently [14,20-22]. Although there is usually a rapid decline in dream recall, if a relatively high incidence persists at a 2-4 hour post-anesthesia interview [11] it is probably a consequence of reinforcement of earlier memories -"new dreams" are infrequent and all dreams are hard to recall, unless actively recalled [23]. New dreams 'during anesthesia' recalled after an initial post-arousal interview may well have occurred between the two interviews. When researching dreaming during anesthesia it is thus important that patients are interviewed immediately after their emergence from anesthesia.

The types of sedative and anesthetic drugs used appear to be an important influence. Sedative drugs alone, for example opioids and benzodiazepines such as midazolam, cause post-procedural dreaming [24]. However the effect of such drugs may be masked when they are used prior to intravenous anesthetic drugs [25].

Scopolamine is a non-selective blocker of muscurinic cholinergic receptors. The CNS cholinergic neurotransmitter system is an important target of general anesthetic drugs. Although used very infrequently (more for its anti-emetic properties than for sedation), the pre-anesthetic administration of scopolamine markedly reduces the incidence of dreaming associated with propofol anesthesia in young women [26]. This may be a consequence of its amnesic effect, which is due to interference with working memory function in the hippocampus.

Antidepressant drugs can alter sleep and dreaming patterns and selective serotonin reuptake inhibitors (SSRIs) may intensify dreaming, especially during acute withdrawal [27], but do not appear to influence dreaming during anesthesia [11].

Propofol is the most widely-used intravenous anesthetic drug and it primarily activates CNS inhibitory neurotransmission via chloride ion channels mediated by the gamma-aminobutyric acid ($GABA_A$) receptor. It also inhibits glutamate activated excitatory neurotransmission and activates cholinergic neurons in the basal forebrain, which are important in the physiology of dream activity [28]. Several observational studies found that induction of anesthesia with propofol, and especially induction and maintenance of anesthesia with propofol, is associated with a higher incidence of dreaming than other methods. Such methods include anesthesia induced with the intravenous barbiturate sodium thiopental (dreaming incidence 7-15% versus 4-45% with propofol) or anesthesia maintained with volatile anesthetic drugs (which are mainly hydroflurocarbons and act at several receptors including $GABA_A$) [20,21,29-35]. A recent large randomized trial found no difference in the incidence of dreaming (approaching 30%) between patients receiving propofol or the inhaled volatile anesthetic desflurane, which results in more rapid recovery from anesthesia than other similar volatile anesthetic drugs [36]. This suggests the propensity for dreaming induced by propofol is not a pharmacodynamic property but due to more rapid recovery associated with propofol than with inhaled volatile anesthetics other than desflurane, which allows verbal assessment of dreaming to take place before a dream is forgotten.

The intravenous anesthetic drug ketamine is a phencyclidine that acts primarily at N-methyl-D-aspartate (NMDA) receptors. It is widely used for general anesthesia in developing countries but rarely used elsewhere, partly because it is associated with delerium due to hallucinations and unpleasant dreams during emergence [37]. Dreaming after ketamine anesthesia is extremely common in young surgical populations (incidence 90%). This can be reduced to 75% by the concurrent administration of a benzodiazepine, although the nature of the dreams is unchanged [38]. Approximately 5-10% of patients find the emergence experience, which typically involves out-of-body (flying or floating) sensations and sometimes transcendental experiences, very disturbing [39,40].

The role of patient factors is less well determined. A study of ketamine and diazepam anesthesia found that neither gender nor age influenced the rate of dreaming [37] and another noted that dreamers were more likely to be male [11]. Nevertheless most studies indicate that women are more likely to report having dreamed [7,10,32,35,41]. This may reflect the fact that women tend to have higher dream recall during sleep [23] and emerge faster from anesthesia than men, so can communicate earlier [35,42].

Dreaming is more common in younger patients [96-11,16,32,35,41], which is consistent with the epidemiology of dreaming during sleep. A large cohort study conducted in children aged 5-12 years found that 10% reported dreaming during anesthesia. There was no association with specific anesthetic drugs but a greater frequency among younger children [22].

Healthier patients experience less sleep disturbance and dream more frequently during anesthesia [9,11,32,35]. Other predictors described include patients having surgery of shorter duration [9,12,30,32] and those having elective rather than emergency surgery [9].

Some studies have found no association between home dreaming and dreaming during anesthesia [26,29,31,32] but there is reasonable evidence for this link [11]. As discussed later, the finding supports the hypothesis that most dreams occur during a pre- or possibly post-arousal sleep state.

Anecdotal reports postulate that steroid-induced psychosis may mimic dreaming [43] and that past or concurrent use of hallucinogenic drugs, such as ecstasy, may predispose to frightening dreams [44].

The Nature and Content of Dreams During Anesthesia and their Sequele

Vivid, distressing or lengthy dreams are not commonly reported after anesthesia [19,29,31,34,45,46]. An example of this type of dream is the narrative "Caving in an old mine. Was pretty cool. Was scary when the lights went out. On the edge of the cave. Lots of colors too. Smell of violets" [11]. Recall of dream content occurs in 75% of those interviewed immediately after they awaken [11] but falls to 10% among patients interviewed later during the recovery phase [9,12,47].

"Hold fast to dreams, for if dreams die, Life is like a broken wing bird that cannot fly" (Langston Hughes). In general patients who report dreaming during anesthesia are also happy they have remembered. After propofol anesthesia only 5-10% of dreams are unpleasant [11,14,15]. Children also report that the content is predominantly pleasant and unrelated to their hospital experience [22].

Propofol usual results in an enjoyable recovery [48]. Compared with thiopentone and volatile anesthetic drugs, intravenous anesthesia with propofol results in mood elevation, positive affect and sensation-seeking tendencies (such as merriment, aggression or enthusiasm) [21,48]. Compared with other anesthetic drugs, patients feel happier during their recovery period [21,29,49] and compared with thiopentone are only half as likely to describe their dreams as unpleasant [12]. Indeed many dreams during anesthesia are described as "very pleasant" and relate to topics such as the family, friends, work or recreational activities [11,16,31,33]. Examples are the following descriptors of dream narratives: "Dreaming of a game of cricket. Was playing with her three children and four grandchildren. She was bowling. She didn't know the oval. It was a beautiful day, a pleasant dream" and "Dreamed she was doing a bridal waltz with her husband – she had been listening to waltz music on the way to the hospital yesterday" [11].

Dreams related to the operation or operating room environment are very uncommon but some may represent 'near-miss' awareness [8,11,12,30,49]. An example of a narrative describing such content is "Described a group of doctors in light blue clothing talking to each other. No sound or perception of touch, movement, pain or paralysis. Did not believe this was related to surgery" [8]. Another example, that quite possibly reflects a memory of the anesthesiologist providing reassurance during an episode of light anesthesia, is the description "Dreaming about driving on a road. The road just swallowed her up. That's it. The doctor said she was Ok but the car was wrecked. She couldn't move – she was trying to tell the driver to stop but he couldn't hear her" [11].

A few patients recall hallucinations or dreams of sexual nature [13,29,50,51]. Most of these reports come from women but male patients probably have similar, but less frequent, sexual hallucinations [13]. There have been several cases in which physicians giving sedation have been charged with sexual assault [50]. Although some such cases may have been genuine, it is now well established that some patients will misconstrue innocuous and trivial events or stimuli (for example applying monitoring devices to the chest) as being of sexual nature, or will experience sexual fantasies. Propofol sedation can result in verbal sexual disinhibition, although use of either propofol or thiopentone does not appear to influence the likelihood of a dream with content related to sex [29]. Indeed a number of studies, involving several hundred patients, have found no cases of erotic dreams or sexual illusions, so this type of dream must occur very infrequently [11,31]. Although in general dreaming is not related to the location or type of surgery and dreams with sexual content may occur irrespective of the type of surgery, in relation to dreams with sexual content the location of the surgery may be a factor. In one study 12% of women displayed amorous and disinhibited behaviour after minor gynecologic surgery under propofol anesthesia, but none did so after abdominal surgery [52]. The anesthesiologist should be aware of these issues and protect themselves against allegations of sexual misconduct, preferably by always remaining chaperoned with a patient of the opposite sex. Allegations should be taken seriously, the patient counselled in the presence of witnesses and meticulous records kept.

Dreaming may affect satisfaction with anesthesia. Leslie et al. [35] found that young women who report dreams after anesthesia were less satisfied with the anesthetic, but this finding was confounded by the presence of higher preoperative anxiety scores in that group. Other studies report that dreaming does not influence satisfaction or anxiety levels in adults [11,21,31] or cause postoperative behavioural disturbance in children [22]. In sedated patients, higher satisfaction with care among dreamers was recently reported [16].

The Timing of Dreaming and its Relationship to Awareness

The association between awareness and dreaming and the fact that dream content very occasionally appears related to the operating environment have led many to conclude that dreaming occurs during periods of "light" anesthesia, when CNS suppression is less profound. This contention is supported by older studies, in which anesthetic techniques that are now considered insufficient because they are confer an unacceptably high incidence of awareness, were also associated with a high frequency of dreaming and of dream content

Table 1. Recent Studies Reporting the Incidence of Dreaming

Patient Population	Year	Interview timing	Incidence	Reference
Non-cardiac surgery and anesthesia including muscle paralysis (n=300)	2009	Immediate	28%	37
Colonoscopy (n = 200)	2008	Immediate	25%	16
All-comers (n = 4001)	2008	PACU	53%	7
Cesarean section (n = 763)	2008	2-6 h, day 2	3%	8
All-comers (n = 6991)	2008	PACU, 1-3 days, 7-14 days	3%	12
BIS monitored (n = 2653)	2008	PACU, 1-3 days, 7-14 days	8%	47
Laparoscopic cholecystectomy and propofol anesthesia (n = 58)	2007	Immediate	10%	55
Atropine, scopolamine preoperatively	2007	Immediate	47%; 0%	26
Anesthesia including muscle paralysis (n = 300)	2007	Immediate	22%	11
Anesthesia including muscle paralysis (n =120)	2006	4-24 h postoperatively	11%	6
Pediatric all-comers (n = 864)	2005	Days 1, 3 and 30	8%, 6%, 5%	22
High risk of awareness (n = 2,453)	2005	2-4 h, 24-36 h, 30 days	4%, 4%, 3%	35
All-comers (n = 19,576)	2004	PACU, 1 week	6%, 3%	9

PACU = post-anesthesia care unit.

related to the operation [14,15,20,31,34,53]. Similarly, women having emergency cesarean section under general anesthetic, a situation associated with a greater risk of awareness than that among the general surgical population, are also more likely to dream than those having elective surgery [54]. With modern approaches to general anesthesia, which more reliably ensure unconsciousness, dream content related to the operating room or hospital environment appears very uncommon [2,11,14,15,29].

Neurophysiological research indicates that patients who report dreaming after anesthesia show higher intraoperative responsiveness of the primary cortex, based on recording of the latency of auditory evoked potentials [54] and raw EEG patterns [37]. Some clinical findings are consistent with the theory that dreaming occurs during light levels of anesthesia, because dreamers receive lower doses of anesthetic drugs than non-dreamers [15,56] and dreamers emerge from the effects of general anesthesia more rapidly [11,35]. Among children, those who experience awareness are also more likely to have dreamed [22] and among adults who dream, the chance of also being aware is much greater (albeit still very infrequent) than among those who don't dream [12]. The incidence of dreams that suggest probable incorporation of auditory memories from a period of light anesthesia is approximately 1 in 300 [11,35]. On the other hand, even dreams apparently clearly indicative of 'near-miss' awareness may subsequently prove to have occurred during recovery from anesthesia, even at a considerable time after leaving the operating area environment and returning to the ward [57].

The alternative theory is that dreaming occurs predominantly during and after emergence from anesthesia, when the patient transitions into a sleep-like state. Drugs which are associated with higher rates of dreaming are those which allow more rapid return of consciousness, for example propofol versus thiopentone and possibly desflurane versus isoflurane. Also, propofol at sub-anaesthetic concentrations does not affect immediate memory recall [58]. Even after sedation (as opposed to anesthesia) with small doses of propofol, midazolam and fentanyl, drowsiness persists for several hours [59]. During sleep onset hallucinations increase in frequency and REM dreams show a parallel increase in bizarre and emotional content. Hypnagogic dreams occur at sleep onset, are truncated, incorporate memories from events of the day or older related memories, and do not show high dream affect, emotion or narrative complexity compared with rapid eye movement (REM) dreams [13]. These characteristics are shared with dreams reported during anesthesia, which are typically short and mundane [11]. In addition, after anesthesia patients are spoken to and stimulated frequently, and dream recall is enhanced when rapid transfer from short-term to long-term memory storage occurs, a process enhanced by higher levels of arousal during sleep [60].

Three recent studies have specifically addressed the question of the timing of dreaming and anesthesia. Leslie et al. tested the hypothesis that dreaming was associated with "light" or inadequate depth of anaesthesia in a prospective cohort study [11]. The hypothesis was rejected – there was no difference between dreamers and non-dreamers in the median values estimating depth of unconsciousness or in the duration of time at which these values were elevated into the range indicative of a greater risk of the return of consciousness. A subsequent and larger study supports these findings [47], even though some patients spent considerable lengths of time at very light levels of anesthesia. Furthermore, no correlation occurred between the depth of anesthesia and the emotional impact of the dream. A large prospective study of almost 7,000 patients found that dream content is similar to that of dreams during sleep and no patient had a dream that subsequently proved to reflect a real intraoperative event [47]. Thus, although patients who dream are many times more likely to also experience awareness than those who don't [12], dreams rarely represent 'near-miss' awareness during the course of anesthesia. Finally, the EEG changes seen in those who dream include increased high frequency power and fewer sleep spindles [37]. This is consistent with EEG patterns during REM-sleep (internal cognitive activity disconnected from external stimuli and associated with reduced responsiveness), although it is not known whether these EEG findings reflect more dreaming mentation or less amnesia for the dreams.

In summary, it appears that most dreams occur when the patient is in a REM-sleep like state during arousal from and in the 5 minutes prior to full wakening from anesthesia.

FUTURE RESEARCH

Dreaming during anesthesia is relatively poorly understood. Does dreaming occur during passage through a physiological sleep plane during emergence from the drug-induced unconsciousness of anesthesia? Although current evidence supports this hypothesis as the likely explanation of the vast majority of dreams during anesthesia, further study of raw EEG data around the time of arousal from anesthesia is needed to look for specific drug-induced effects This information would help to further clarify the nature of EEG activity during light anesthesia, arousal from unconsciousness and initial post-arousal sedation, compared with that during phases of sleep.

Apart from ketamine, which causes distinctive emergence reactions and dreams, it remains uncertain whether different pharmacologic effects of anesthetic drugs significantly influence dreaming or whether confounding factors, including the speed of emergence from unconsciousness, explain most of the reported variability.

CONCLUSION

A patient who postoperatively recalls actual intraoperative events during general anesthesia has been conscious and is described as having been “aware”. Dreaming during anesthesia has been defined as any other recalled experience that occurred between induction of general anesthesia and the first return of consciousness after anesthesia. Although it is described by up to 50% of patients, the incidence is dependent not only on the timing of the post-anesthesia interview but also on a number of patient and anesthetic characteristics.

The dream content is often recalled but is typically limited in scope, related to everyday events, emotionally neutral or pleasant and free of harmful consequences. Rarely, the dream content suggests a ‘near-miss’ awareness experience that resulted from an inadequate depth of anesthesia. Most dreams appear to occur during a sleep state, similar to REM sleep, in the period immediately prior to initial arousal from unconsciousness at the end of anesthesia, but this requires further evaluation.

REFERENCES

[1] Bruhn, J; Myles, PS; Sneyd, R; Struys, MMRF. Depth of anaesthesia monitoring: what’s available, what’s validated and what’s next? *Br J Anaesth,* 2006;97:85-94

[2] Myles, PS; Leslie, K; McNeil, J; Forbes, A; Chan, MTV; for the B-Aware trial group. Bispectral index monitoring to prevent awareness during anaesthesia: the B-Aware randomised controlled trial. *The Lancet,* 2004;363:1757-1763.

[3] Hobson, J. *Dreaming: An Introduction to the Science of Sleep.* Oxford: Oxford University Press; 2002.

[4] Lubke, GH; Kerssens, C; Gershon, RY; Sebel, PS. Memory formation during general anesthesia for emergency cesarean section. *Anesthesiology,* 2000;92:1029-1034.

[5] Nordstrom, O; Sandin, R. Recall during intermittent propofol anaesthesia. *Br J Anaesth,* 1996;76:699-701.

[6] Stonell, CA; Leslie, K; He, C; Lee, L. No sex differences in memory formation during general anesthesia. *Anesthesiology*, 2006;105:920-926.

[7] Errando, CL; Sigl, JC; Robles, M; Calabuig, E; Garcia, J; Arocas, F; Higueras, R; Del Rosario, E; Lopez, D; Peiro, CM; Soriano, JL; Chaves, S; Gil, F; Garcia-Aguado, R. Awareness with recall during general anaesthesia: a prospective observational evaluation of 4001 patients. *Br J Anaesth*, 2008;101:178-185.

[8] Paech, MJ; Scott, KL; Clavisi, O; Chua, S; McDonnell, N; the ANZCA Trials Group. A prospective study of awareness and recall associated with general anaesthesia for caesarean section. *Int J Obstet Anesth*, 2008;17:298-303.

[9] Sebel, PS; Bowdle, TA; Ghoneim, MM; Rampil, IJ; Padilla, RE; Gan, TJ; Domino, KB. The incidence of awareness during anesthesia: a multicenter study United States study. *Anesth Analg,* 2004;99:833-839.

[10] Ranta, SOV; Laurila, R; Saario, J; Ali-Melkkila, T; Hynynen, M. Awareness with recall during general anesthesia: incidence and risk factors. *Anesth Analg,* 1998;86:1084-1089.

[11] Leslie, K; Skrzypek, H; Paech, MJ; Kurowski, I; Whybrow, T. Dreaming during anesthesia and anesthetic depth in elective surgical patients. A prospective cohort study. *Anesthesiology,* 2007;106:33-42.

[12] Samuelsson, P; Brudin, L; Sandin, RH. Intraoperative dreams reported after general anaesthesia are not early interpretations of delayed awareness. *Acta Anaesthesiol Scand,* 2008;52:805-809.

[13] Strickland, RA; Butterworth, JF. Sexual dreaming during anesthesia. Early case histories (1849-1888) of the phenomenon. *Anesthesiology*, 2007;106:1232-1236.

[14] Brice, DD; Hetherington, RR; Utting, JE. A simple study of awareness and dreaming during anaesthesia. *Br J Anaesth*, 1970;42:535-541.

[15] Harris, TJB; Brice, DD; Hetherington, RR; Utting, JE. Dreaming associated with anaesthesia: the influence of morphine premedication and two volatile adjuvants. *Br J Anaesth,* 1971;43:172-178.

[16] Stait, ML; Leslie, K; Bailey, R. Dreaming and recall during sedation for colonoscopy. *Anaesth Intensive Care*, 2008;36:685-690.

[17] Scheman, JD; Gottlieb, A; Spring J. Flashback and nightmares after surgery under neuraxial anesthesia: a report of two cases. *Arch Phys Med Rehabil* 1998;79:579-581.

[18] Hunter, DN; Thonley, A; Whitburn, R. Arousal from propofol. *Anaesthesia,* 1987;42:1128-1129.

[19] Young, PN. Hallucinations after propofol. *Anaesthesia*, 1988;43:170.

[20] Marsch, SCU; Schaefer, HG; Tschan, C; Meier, B. Dreaming and anaesthesia: total i.v. anaesthesia with propofol versus balanced volatile anaesthesia with enflurane. *Euro J Anaesthesiol,* 1992;9:331-333.

[21] Oxorn, D; Orser, B; Ferris, LE; Harrington, E. Propofol and thiopentone anesthesia: a comparison of the incidence of dreams and perioperative mood alterations. *Anesth Analg*, 1994;79:553-557.

[22] Huang, GH; Davidson, AJ; Stargatt, R. Dreaming during anaesthesia in children: incidence, nature and associations. *Anaesthesia,* 2005;60:854-861.
[23] Schredl, M. Questionnaires and diaries as research instruments in dream research: methodological issues. *Dreaming*, 2002;12:17-26.
[24] Swann, A; Williams, J; Fatovich, DM. Recall after procedural sedation in the emergency department. *Emerg Med J,* 2007;24:322-324.
[25] Oxorn, DC; Ferris, LE; Harrington, E; Orser, BA. The effects of midazolam on propofol-induced anesthesia: propofol dose requirements, mood profiles, and perioperative dreams. *Anesth Analg*, 1997;85:553-559.
[26] Toscano, A ; Pancaro, C ; Peduto, VA. Scopolamine prevents dreams during general anesthesia. *Anesthesiology,* 2007;106:952-955.
[27] Pace-Schott, EF; Gersh, T; Silverstri, R; Stickgold, R; Salzman, C; Hobson, JA. SSRI treatment suppresses dream recall frequency but increases subjective dream intensity in normal subjects. *J Sleep Res*, 2001;10:129-142.
[28] Stickgold, R; Hobson, JA; Fosse, R; Fosse, M. Sleep, learning, and dreams: Off-line memory reprocessing. *Science,* 2001;294:1052-1057.
[29] Brandner, B; Blagrove, M; McCallum, G; Bromley, LM. Dreams, images and emotions associated with propofol anaesthesia. *Anaesthesia*, 1997;52:750-755.
[30] Smyth, DG; Collins-Howgill, PJ. Hallucinations after propofol. *Anaesthesia*, 1998;43:170.
[31] Hellwagner, K; Holzer, A; Gustorff, B; Schroegendorfer, K; Greher, M; Weindlmayr-Goettel, M; Saleru, B; Lackner, FX. Recollection of dreams after short general anaesthesia: influence on patient anxiety and satisfaction. *Euro J Anaesthesiol*, 2003;20:282-288.
[32] Kasmacher, H; Petermeyer, M; Decker, C. Incidence and quality of dreaming during anesthesia with propofol in comparison with enflurane. *Anaesthesist,* 1996;45:146-153.
[33] Gunawardene, RD. Propofol and dreaming. *Anaesthesia*, 1989;44:266-267.
[34] Ghoneim , MM; Block, RI; Dhanaraj, VJ; Todd, MM; Choi, WW; Brown, CK. Auditory evoked responses and learning and awareness during general anaesthesia. *Acta Anaesthesiol Scand,* 2000;44:133-143.
[35] Leslie, K; Myles, PS; Forbes, A; Chan, MTV; Swallow, SK; Short, TG. Dreaming during anaesthesia in patients at high risk of awareness. *Anaesthesia,* 2005;60:239-244.
[36] Wanna, O; Werawatganon, T; Piriyakitphaiboon, S; Taesiri, B. A comparison of propofol and ketamine as induction agents for caesarean section. *J Med Assoc Thai,* 2004;87:774-779.
[37] Leslie, K; Sleigh, J; Paech, MJ; Voss, L; Lim, CW; Sleigh, C. Dreaming and electroencephalographic changes during anesthesia maintained with propofol or desflurane. *Anesthesiology,* 2009;111:547-555.
[38] Grace, RF. The effect of variable-dose diazepam on dreaming and emergence phenomena in 400 cases of ketamine-fentanyl anaesthesia. *Anaesthesia,* 2003;58:904-910.
[39] Morgan, M; Loh, L. Ketamine as the sole anaesthetic agent for minor surgical procedures. *Anaesthesia*, 1971;26:158-165.
[40] Hostetler, MA; Davis, CO. Prospective age-based comparison of behavioural reactions occurring after ketamine sedation in the ED. *Am J Emerg Med*, 2002;20:463-468.

[41] Wilson, SL; Vaughan, RW; Stephen, CR. Awareness, dreams, hallucinations associated with general anesthesia. *Anesth Analg,* 1975; 54:609-617.

[42] Myles, P; Hunt, J; Fletcher, H. Sex differences in speed of emergence and quality of recovery after anaesthesia: A cohort study. *Br Med J*, 2001;322;710-711.

[43] Hayward, E; Healy, D; Wimbush, S. Awareness, dreaming or steroid-induced psychosis? *Anaesthesia,* 2006;61:1116-1129.

[44] Morris, GN; Magee, PT. Anaesthesia and past use of LSD. *Can J Anaesth*, 1995;42:177-179.

[45] Millar, JM; Jewkes, CF. Recovery and morbidity after daycase anaesthesia. *Anaesthesia*, 1988;43:738-743.

[46] Suresh, D. Nightmares and recovery from anesthesia. *Anesth Analg,* 1991;72:404-405.

[47] Samuelsson, P; Brudin, L; Sandin, RH. BIS does not predict dreams reported after anaesthesia. *Acta Anaesthesiol Scand*, 2008;52:810-814.

[48] Zacny, JP; Lichtor, JL; Thompson, W; Apfelbaum, JL. Propofol at a subanesthetic dose may have abuse potential. *Anesth Analg*, 1993;77:544-552.

[49] Oddby-Muhrbeck, E; Jakobsson, J. Recall of music: a comparison between anaesthesia with propofol and isoflurane. *Acta Anaesthesiol Scand*, 1993;37:33-37.

[50] Balasubramaniam, B; Park, GR. Sexual hallucinations during and after sedation and anaesthesia. *Anaesthesia*, 2003;58:549-553.

[51] Kent, EA; Bacon, DR; Harrison, P; Lema, MJ. Sexual illusions and propofol sedation. *Anesthesiology,* 1992;77:1037-1038.

[52] Bricker, SRW. Hallucinations after propofol. *Anaesthesia,* 1988;43:171.

[53] McKie, BD; Thorp, EA. Awareness and dreaming during anaesthesia in a paediatric hospital. *Anaesth Intensive Care,* 1973;1:407-414.

[54] Bogod, DG; Orton, JK; Yau, HM; Oh, TE. Detecting awareness during general anaesthetic Caesarean section. An evaluation of two methods. *Anaesthesia,* 1990;45:279-284.

[55] Aceto, P; Congedo, E; Lai, C; Valente, A; Gualtieri, E; De Cosmo, G. Dreams recall and auditory evoked potentials during propofol anaesthesia. *Neuroreport,* 2007;18:823-826.

[56] Latto, I; Waldron, B. Anaesthesia for caesarean section: analysis of blood concentrations of halothane using 0.2% or 0.65% halothane with 50% nitrous oxide in oxygen. *Br J Anaesth,* 1977;49:371-378.

[57] Adams, H. Awareness, dreaming or steroid-induced psychosis. *Anaesthesia,* 2007;62:198.

[58] Zacny, JP; Lichtor, JL; Coalson, DW; Finn, RS; Uitvlugt, AM; Glosten, B; Flemming, DC; Apfelbaum, JL. Subjective and psychomotor effects of subanesthetic doses of propofol in healthy volunteers. *Anesthesiology,* 1992;76:696-702.

[59] Lichtor, JL; Alessi, R; Lane, BS. Sleep tendency as a measure of recovery after drugs used for ambulatory surgery. *Anesthesiology*, 2002;96:878-883.

[60] Goodenough, DR. Dream recall: history and current status of the field. In: Ellman SJ, Antrobus JS editors. *The Mind in Sleep*. New York: Wiley; 1991; 143-171.

In: Psychiatric Research Trends: Dreams and Geriatric Psychiatry ISBN 978-1-60741-760-6
Editors: Daniella M. Montez, pp.145-150

Chapter 9

Educational Opportunities in the Study of Dreams and Dreaming

*W. Jeff Bryson**
Department of Psychology, Jacksonville State University, Jacksonville, AL, USA and School of Psychology, Fielding Graduate University, Santa Barbara, CA, USA

General Academic and Community Education

The study of dreams and dreaming represents an important area of knowledge that spans many academic disciplines including anthropology, cognitive science, consciousness science, medicine, neuroscience, philosophy, psychology, and sociology. Still, it is uncommon to find a formal course or program that is specific to dreams at the undergraduate, graduate, and postgraduate levels despite the broad application of this subject across so many fields of study. Statistical information regarding academic courses or programs that provide at least a major component on the subject of dreaming among each discipline has not been well documented. Community education on dreaming also appears to be quite scarce. Educational materials on dreams and dreaming are also available online, although these materials are certainly not well regulated. This renders a problem in that it would be difficult for many lay persons to differentiate appropriate versus unsubstantiated content, leading to a potentially negative influence on general public knowledge. There are certainly many challenges that remain for the future of educational opportunities in the area of dreams and dreaming that need to be addressed.

Literature on the topic of dream-specific education is available, albeit scarce. Frank and Trunell (1978) described an experiential method for teaching dream synthesis to candidate psychoanalysts. Ullman (1994) also noted a pedagogic method for training therapists. Krippner, Gabel, Green, and Rubien (1994) discussed methods for teaching dreamwork in community programs. Recent efforts have been made to revive the development of coursework and pedagogic techniques specific to the study of dreams and dreaming (Bryson,

* Contact: Jeff Bryson, Department of Psychology, Jacksonville State University, 700 Pelham Road, North, Jacksonville, Alabama, 36265, USA. Email: jbryson@jsu.edu

2002, 2003; Bryson, Kinsey, Mastin, and Bryson, 2009; Bryson, Mastin, Pilgreen, and Bryson, 2008). Although published literature on dream education is not necessary for expanding opportunities, it does reflect the scarcity of available courses specific to this subject matter.

Dreaming is sometimes covered in the context of broader coursework. For example, courses such as introductory level psychology cover a brief overview of major dream theories and characteristics (Bryson et al., 2009). Academic courses such as those taught on the subject of sleep also provide an excellent environment for covering expanded dream content (Bryson, 2002, 2003; Bryson et al., 2009; Bryson et al., 2008). A specific pedagogic exercise available in this context is Dream Lab (Bryson, 2002, 2003; Bryson et al., 2009; Bryson et al., 2008). Dream Lab is an experiential model for teaching both dream theories and characteristics. This exercise is particularly useful in that it is designed to be applicable as a supplement to a variety of courses regardless of academic discipline (Bryson et al., 2009; Bryson et al., 2008). The specific theories and characteristics could also be customized depending on the needs of the course. Using this technique in a workshop or continuing education format has not been formally explored but is certainly encouraged.

Future efforts to extend educational opportunities in all areas are certainly needed. It is important to recognize that there are relatively few scientists that focus their studies and careers on dreaming. It is certainly possible to expand the availability of dream-specific educational opportunities in the general academic and community settings, although this responsibility will ultimately fall on the shoulders of current dream scientists and philosophers. Several areas need to be addressed for expansion of educational opportunities to occur. This includes the development of new coursework, course supplements, community outreach, and online resources. Each of these presents unique challenges to the dream educator.

Efforts to expand dream-specific educational opportunities at all academic levels are desirable. Expanding opportunities at the undergraduate level are particularly recommended. This is because exposing students at earlier stages in their academic careers serves as a potential means for recruiting new scientists into the field. Formal training and education at the graduate and postgraduate levels are also needed to support the development of new scientists interested in careers in the area of dreams.

Creating new courses at all levels of higher education often involves a great deal of effort and a degree of opportunity. Courses designed to address the topic of dreams and dreaming would most likely serve as an elective rather than a requirement. This presents an issue of necessity in that these courses would be of academic value, but may not be considered essential in most programs. Also, as mentioned earlier, there are relatively few professionals that have a major interest in the subject of dreams. Further, those employed in an academic setting often have preexisting obligations to certain courses. Here, adding a course will potentially surpass the instructor's limitations and, thus, limit the creation and instruction of a new course. There must also be a willingness or need on the part of the academic institution to expand coursework. These opportunities are likely to be presented in brief windows and would occur periodically every so many years or even decades. Clearly, the recipe for creating a new dream-specific course involves a combination of having a professor available to create and teach the course, as well as an academic institution that is ready and open to the creation of that course. Future expansion of such courses in formal education settings depends on willing professors to be prepared to take advantage of these opportunities when the conditions are favorable.

Course supplementation of dream-specific materials is often easier to accomplish when the subject of dreams is integral to the broader course. Here, developing ways to enhance the quality of dream-related content is often at the discretion of the instructor. While there is no formula for enhancing this type of education, each instructor must challenge themselves to provide a presentation of the material in a way that maximizes student knowledge and interest.

Dream-specific community education programs are not as likely to become widespread due to the ease and speed to which people can access information online. If developed, these programs would most likely thrive in populous areas where small groups of people were interested in personal enrichment taught in an interactive environment and in the presence of a live instructor. On a global scale, developing an online versus live workshop would also likely depend on the culture and availability of various media resources.

Online resources related to dreams and dreaming is abundant but, again, hit or miss in terms of quality. Unfortunately, it is impossible to delete all misinformative sites from the internet. It is important, however, to ensure that quality educational websites are available to the public. Developing informative sites sponsored by universities or organizations offers visitors interested in quality personal enrichment some sense of credibility. It is also recommended that these sites offer references and suggested reading material so that these individuals have the opportunity to verify content or pursue further education if they choose.

The expansion of general academic and community education on the subject of dreams is quite possible with some effort. Present and future dream educators are encouraged to take advantage of opportunities to promote this expansion whenever possible. Providing education in terms of academic settings and in the community is a means to expand genral knowledge of dreams to a broader population. Another avenue that will require some attention is providing education and training opportunities to those involved in the delivery of clinical services.

EDUCATION FOR CLINICAL APPLICATIONS

Working with dreams in the course of therapeutic intervention is certainly not a new concept for psychiatrists and clinical psychologists. Psychoanalysis recognized the value of dreams for this purpose over a century ago (Freud, 1900). Other approaches such as Jungian (analytical), Adlerian (individual), and Gestalt psychotherapies have also embraced the importance of dreams as part of the overall therapeutic process (Douglas, 2008; Hill, 1996; Mosak and Maniacci, 2008). Cognitive-behavioral therapies (CBT), in general, have been less reliant on incorporating dream content compared to many of the other approaches. This, however, does not negate the merit of using dreams in the course of CBT. Here, many therapists trained in CBT are simply not provided with a strong background for understanding dreams and the applicability of this content to the therapeutic process (Crook, 2004; Freeman and White, 2002). Furthermore, empirical research on the applicability of dreams in the therapeutic milieu has been a particular challenge for all theoretical orientations. CBT is strongly dependent upon empirical validation and the inherent challenges of clinical dream research have thus far been extensively avoided in this orientation. Dreams are, however, representative phenomena of human existence and cannot be discounted by any theoretical approach. Therefore, therapists are strongly encouraged to gain an understanding of dreams and the applicability of these experiences regardless of his or her chosen style of therapy. Although dream education is encouraged for all therapists, enhancing the ability to work with dreams among those providing CBT is a particularly important area of need.

Dreams were addressed in the early formulations of cognitive therapy (Beck, 1971). This theoretical development was, for the most part, abandoned and left dormant for much of the past four decades (Rosner, 2004). Fortunately, there has been a much needed resurgence in attention given to dreaming among CBT practitioners in recent years (Rosner, Lyddon, and Freeman, 2004). It is hopeful that this will lead to further research in developing a theoretical basis for incorporating dreams into CBT and an opportunity to improve educational programs for cognitive therapists.

Choosing to work with dreams in the course of psychotherapy is often at the discretion of the therapist. Furthermore, working with dreams in this context is not necessarily restricted to a particular form of psychopathology. Individuals may present therapists with dream content at any time during the course of his or her treatment. In some cases, however, dreams may be a primary target for the intervention. The approach to treating this will, of course, depend on type of therapy being provided. From the CBT standpoint, one specific technique developed to address disturbing dreams and nightmares is imagery rehearsal therapy (IRT; Krakow, Kellner, Neidhardt, Pathak, and Lambert, 1993; Krakow, Kellner, Pathak; and Lambert, 1995). IRT is, unfortunately, still a form of psychotherapy that is not necessarily present in the repertoire of many CBT practitioners. The ability to provide this particular intervention strategy, however, is likely to be a useful resource for many therapists given the likelihood of encountering patients who have been exposed to various psychological traumas.

Those prescribing medications also have a need for education with respect to dreaming. An extensive search of the literature in any medical library database will reveal a plethora of pharmacological agents that have the potential to alter dreaming. This will, inevitably, be concerning for some patients and it is important that the clinician be prepared to deal with these concerns as they arise. Providing physicians with preparation for dealing with this can be brief as long as the education provides a sufficient resource for promoting patient reassurance and facilitating compliance with needed treatments.

The current levels to which various training programs for psychiatrists and clinical psychologists cover dreaming is difficult to ascertain. This would certainly depend on the type of theoretical orientation held by the program and the specific curriculum of the individual program itself. Creating opportunities to study dreams is an important clinical endeavor at all levels of education and training. Providing clinicians with a greater exposure to dreams is expected to spark research interests in some, which will, in turn, benefit the field well into the future. Still, improving research on the applicability of dreams in the therapeutic setting is a worthwhile and, yet, formidable challenge to clinical scientists. For now, training workshops on clinical aspects of dreaming are most likely to be presented at scientific meetings. Clinicians at all levels of training and professional practice interested in working with dreams are strongly encouraged to seek out and attend these training opportunities.

Conclusions and Future Direction

The future of dreams and dreaming as a topic of study is promising. There is a tremendous need to develop educational opportunities that will reach a large portion of the population. Developing training for clinicians to work with dreams in the treatment setting is another area of particular need. It will be a tremendous challenge to expand educational opportunities in all areas of this field. With that said, it is important that educational opportunities be expanded and maintained as a means of supporting the field of dream studies well into the future.

References

Beck, A. T. (1971). Cognitive patterns in dreams and daydreams. In J. H. Masserman (Ed.), *Dream dynamics: Science and psychoanalysis* (Vol. 19, pp. 2-7). New York: Grune and Stratton.

Bryson, W. J. (2002). New curriculum benefits undergraduate psychology students. *Sleep Review, 3*(4), 10-12.

Bryson, W. J. (2003). Learning on the web. *Sleep Review, 4*(5), 10-14.

Bryson, W. J., Kinsey, C., Mastin, D. F., and Bryson, T. L. (2009). Dream Lab for introductory psychology. *North American Journal of Psychology, 11*, 353-360.

Bryson, W. J., Mastin, D. F., Pilgreen, K. L., and Bryson, T. L. (2008). Dream Lab: An experiential pedagogic approach to dream theories and characteristics. *Dreaming, 18,* 122-126.

Crook, R. E. (2004). A comparison of cognitive, psychodynamic, and eclectic therapists' attitudes and practices in working with dreams in psychotherapy. In R. I. Rosner, W. J. Lyddon, and A. Freeman (Eds.) *Cognitive therapy and dreams* (pp. 33-53). New York: Springer.

Douglas, C. (2008). Analytical psychotherapy. In R. J. Corsini and D. Wedding (Eds.) *Current psychotherapies* (8th ed., pp. 107-139). Belmont, CA: Thompson Brooks/Cole.

Freeman, A., and White, B. (2002). Dreams and the dream image: Using dreams in cognitive therapy. *Journal of Cognitive Psychotherapy, 16*, 39-53.

Freud, S. (1900). *Die traumdeutung*. Leipzig and Vienna: Franz Deuticke.

Frank, A., and Trunnell, E. E. (1978). Conscious dream synthesis as a method of learning about dreaming: A pedagogic experiment. *Psychoanalytic Quarterly, 47*, 103-112.

Hill, C. E. (1996). *Working with dreams in psychotherapy*. New York: The Guilford Press.

Krakow, B., Kellner, R., Neidhardt, J., Pathak, D., and Lambert, L. (1993). Imagery rehearsal treatment of chronic nightmares: With a thirty month follow-up. *Journal of Behavior Therapy and Experimental Psychiatry, 24*, 325-330.

Krakow, B., Kellner, R., Pathak, D., and Lambert, L. (1995). Imagery rehearsal treatment for chronic nightmares. *Behaviour Research and Therapy, 33*, 837-843.

Kripner, S., Gabel, S., Green, J., and Rubien, R. (1994). Community applications of an experiential group approach to teaching dreamwork. *Dreaming, 4*, 215-222.

Mosak, H. H., and Maniacci, M. P. (2008). Adlerian psychotherapy. In R. J. Corsini and D. Wedding (Eds.) *Current psychotherapies* (8th ed., pp. 63-102). Belmont, CA: Thompson Brooks/Cole.

Rosner, R. I. (2004). Aaron T. Beck's dream theory in context: An introduction to his 1971 article on cognitive patterns in dreams and daydreams. In R. I. Rosner, W. J. Lyddon, and A. Freeman (Eds.) *Cognitive therapy and dreams* (pp. 9-26). New York: Springer.

Rosner, R. I., Lyddon, W. J., and Freeman, A. (2004). Cognitive therapy and dreams: An introduction. In R. I. Rosner, W. J. Lyddon, and A. Freeman (Eds.) *Cognitive therapy and dreams* (pp. 3-8). New York: Springer.

Ullman, M. (1994). The experiential dream group: Its application in the training of therapists. *Dreaming, 4*, 223-229.

In: Psychiatric Research Trends: Dreams and Geriatric Psychiatry ISBN 978-1-60741-760-6
Editors: Daniella M. Montez, pp.151-169

Chapter 10

LUCID DREAMING: A NEURAL SIMULATION OF THE REAL WORLD

Daniel Erlacher*
University of Heidelberg, Germany

1. INTRODUCTION

Dreams can be considered as a kind of simulation of the real world on a higher cognitive level (Erlacher & Schredl, 2008b). In a dream the dreamer experiences himself as a dream ego within a dream environment. The dream ego can either actively take part in the plot or observe the ongoing dream. The content of dreams can be very diverse regarding a variety of characteristics, ranging from bizarre to realistic, negative to positive emotions, emotional to rational elements, and so on (cf. Schredl & Wittmann, 2005). After awaking from a dream people often state that they perceived their experience within the dream in a similar way as they might have during wakefulness (Schredl & Hofmann, 2003). A simple explanation for the fact that dreams often seem to mimic the real world so perfectly is that the neural processes of the brain which underlie the dream simulation are the same processes that occur during wakefulness (Schredl, 2000). This notion is underlined by the fact that during REM sleep – the sleep state during which most vivid dreaming occurs – the EEG recording shows high activity of the brain in contrast to NREM sleep (Hobson, Pace-Schott, & Stickgold, 2000). Research applying modern imaging tools (PET, fMRI) shows that the dreaming brain reveals for specific brain areas activations similar to wakefulness whereas other areas tend to be inactive (Dang-Vu et al., 2005). Additionally, the specific activation of the brain corresponds to the specific characteristic of the dream experience, e.g. high activity in the visual association cortex causes visual hallucinosis during dreaming (Hobson et al., 2000). In this paper, therefore, I will assume that especially during REM sleep the brain produces a perfect simulation of the real world on a higher cognitive level.

---

* Corresponding author: Daniel Erlacher, PhD, Institute of Sports and Sport Sciences, Heidelberg University, Im Neuenheimer Feld 700, 69120 Heidelberg, Germany, Email: Daniel.erlacher@issw.uni-heidelberg.de, Phone: +49 (6221) 54-4348, Fax: +49 (6221) 54-4387

A special kind of nocturnal dreams is lucid dreaming. In a lucid dream the dreamer realizes the dream state and he or she is often able to control the dream simulation and do whatever he or she wants to do. Because the phenomenon of lucid dreaming seems to be hard to grasp, the first part of the paper will focus on several basic aspects of lucid dreaming. The dreaming brain seems to be an excellent choice to study the relationship between the subjective level and the physiological level. In the second part of the paper psychophysiological studies on lucid dreaming will be reviewed. Those studies do support my assumption that the dreaming brain indeed reflects a simulated world on a higher level. In the third part of the paper different applications of lucid dreaming will be discussed. As a final point, some further future directions for lucid dream research will be presented.

2. General Findings About Lucid Dreaming

2.1. What Is the Definition of a Lucid Dream?

Before trying to define what a lucid dream is, we need to agree on a general definition of dreaming. The following definition is widely accepted:

> "A dream or dream report is the recollection of mental activity which has occurred during sleep." (Schredl, 1999, p. 12)

It is important to notice that a dream is not objectively recordable. It is possible to record the physiology of the sleeping body (e.g. respiration, brain activity) with modern recording devices and this data can be analyzed; however, one's experience while dreaming is only accessible for the dreamer. In dream research, therefore, it is important to separate the physiological level from the psychological level (Schredl, 1999). In order to obtain a dream report from a participant in dream studies, two limitations have to be considered: First, the sleep/wake transition and, second, the recollection of the dream for which the time between the dream occurrence and the recollection of the dream is crucial. If the dreamer awakens directly from the dream the chance to recall more of the dream is higher than when the dreamer recalls the dream several hours after the dream (Schredl & Reinhard, 2008a). The mentioned problems for the definition of a dream are also relevant for the definition of a lucid dream (Erlacher & Schredl, 2008b).

In the literature about lucid dreaming several definitions for a lucid dream can be found. All definitions have one particular criterion in common, which is that a lucid dream is a dream in which the dreamer – while dreaming – is aware that she/he is dreaming (cf. Schredl & Erlacher, 2004). This minimum criterion is widely accepted. Depending on the author different additional criteria have to be met in order for a dream to be considered a lucid dream. Tholey (1988), for example, proposed the following additional criteria:

1. Clarity regarding one's own ability to decide to do something
2. Clarity with regard to recollecting one's waking life, especially to recollecting what one intended to investigate in the dream
3. Clarity respecting recollecting the dream after awakening

Tholey's third criterion refers to the fact that after awakening only the recalled dreams can be reported (Schredl, 1999). Considering that after each night only a limited number of dreams can be recalled, it seems plausible that this is also true for lucid dreams (Erlacher, 2007). The first two criterions have been most discussed. Tart (1984), for example, argued that the minimal criterion is not sufficient for the definition of a lucid dream because the feeling of knowing that one is dreaming is a rather common phenomenon but to control the dream and to remember the waking memories is the unique feature of lucid dreaming. Furthermore, Tart (1984), proposed to differentiate between lucid dreams and dreaming-awareness dreams. With the term lucid dream Tart defines dreams in which the "dreamer is aware that he is dreaming, clearly recalls his waking life, and considers himself to be in full command of his intellectual and motivational abilities" (p. 5). On the other hand, he proposes the term "dreaming-awareness dreams" to describe dreams that include some concurrent awareness that one is dreaming, but where this awareness is not accompanied by a shift in consciousness to the altered state of lucid dreaming.

Gillespie (1984) argued that a distinction between lucid dreaming and dreaming-awareness dreams would cause a number of problems. One dilemma is that the additional criteria need to be operationalized. A study by Barrett (1992) demonstrates this problem. In her study she rated 49 lucid dreams with four different corollaries: 1) People in dreams are dream characters, 2) Dream objects are not real, i.e., actions will not carry over concretely upon awakening, 3) The dreamer does not need to obey waking-life physics to achieve a goal, 4) Memory of the waking world is intact rather than amnesic or fictitious. Results showed that only about half of the dream reports were lucid for any particular corollary and less than a 25% could be considered lucid regarding all four characteristics. Beside those results the study revealed methodological problems of dream content analysis. Dream research shows, that the subjective dream experience and the objective dream rating is not always valid (Schredl & Erlacher, 2003). With respect to the mentioned methodological problems, I will prefer in this paper the straightforward definition of a lucid dream, which defines lucid dreams as dreams in which the dreamer is aware of the dreaming state (see also Erlacher, 2009).

2.2. When do Lucid Dreams Occur?

Lucid dreaming is a phenomenon of the sleeping brain; however, the question arises which sleep stage is related to lucid dreaming. To answer this question some general aspects of sleep have to be considered first. Sleep has long been seen as a passive state in which the body and brain recovers from daytime activity. In recent years it became apparent that the sleeping brain is never inactive; rather, specific brain regions are activated more or less throughout the night (e.g. Hobson & Pace-Schott, 2002). REM (rapid eye movement) sleep is a sleep stage in which the brain has high activation (Dang-Vu et al., 2005). This state occurs in approximately 90-100 minute cycles, alternating with four stages of quiescent sleep known as non-REM sleep (Rechtschaffen & Kales, 1968). During a normal night of sleep a person, therefore, will have between 4 to 6 REM sleep periods. The duration of REM periods gets longer during the second half of the night, whereas slow wave sleep is predominant during the first half of the night. The high activation of the brain during REM sleep can be linked to the high percentage of vivid dreams which normal subjects report after awakening from REM sleep. In contrast to the high activation of the dreaming brain the physical body is nearly paralyzed because the efferent motor commands are actively suppressed by neural structures in the brain stem (Hobson et al., 2000). This mechanism is important because it keeps the dreamer from actually acting out his or her dream.

Already back in the 1960's an early study from Dement and Kleitman (1957a) demonstrated that up to 80 % of participants that were awaken from REM sleep remembered a vivid dream whereas only 20 % of participants woken up during NREM sleep could report a dream. Even though later studies showed that dreams during NREM sleep can occur more often, dreams during REM sleep are considered more intensive in quantity and quality (cf. Hobson et al., 2000).

How can lucid dreams be validated when the sleeping body is paralyzed and a direct communication between the dreamer and the researcher is not possible. The answer is that the paralysis of the skeletal muscles during REM sleep has one obvious exception: Rapid Eye Movements. The REMs observed in a sleeping person in part do correspond to the eye movements done by the dreamer (cf. Roffwarg, Dement, Muzio, & Fischer, 1962). This fact can be used in sleep laboratory studies where lucid dreamers can execute pre-agreed and specific eye movements to mark events in the recordings of the electrooculogram (EOG). With this method a strong correlation between lucid dreamed actions and physiological measurements (e.g. EEG, EMG, hear rate) was found (see chapter on "psychophysiological relationship during lucid dreams"). Those studies support the notion that lucid dreams occur almost exclusively in REM dreams.

2.3. How Many People Have Lucid Dreams?

The question about how many people have lucid dreams has two aspects to it: How many people have ever had at least one lucid dream (prevalence) and how often do lucid dreamers have lucid dreams (frequency). Regarding the first question a representative survey in Austria (N = 1000) found that 26% of participants stated they had experienced at least one a lucid dream (Stepansky et al., 1998). For university student samples, the figures are markedly higher and range from 47% to 92% (cf. Erlacher, Schredl, Watanabe, Yamana, & Ganzert, 2008). Snyder and Gackenbach (1988) reported results from seven further surveys with prevalence rates ranging from 47% to 100% (e.g., members of a dream seminar).

The high variability in the prevalence of lucid dreaming can be explained by sampling procedures (e.g., random vs. representative samples). A further factor to consider might be the presence of a definition of lucid dreaming or an example of a lucid dream within the questionnaire to avoid that participants might misunderstand the phenomenon. In some studies participant were asked for additional verification of the lucid dream. Participants had to report a recent lucid dream example which was then rated by a trained judge as being either lucid or non-lucid. In general, the prevalence becomes smaller for samples with a verification of lucid dreams and a definition or an example within the questionnaire (cf. Snyder & Gackenbach, 1988).

Regarding the second aspect, lucid dream frequency, Snyder and Gackenbach (1988) classified participants in frequent lucid dreamers with one or more lucid dreams per month and infrequent lucid dreamers with less than one lucid dream per month (but a least one lucid dream). Here several surveys have shown that the percentages of frequent lucid dreamers range from 17% to 36%.

Only a few studies have measured the frequency of lucid dreaming by counting the number of lucid dreams in a dream diary. The percentage of lucid dreams from the total amount of recalled dreams within a dream diary ranges from 0.3% to 0.7% for non-lucid dreamers and for lucid dreamers the percentage of lucid dreams from the total amount of recalled dreams is 17.3% (Zadra, Donderi, & Pihl, 1992).

Two studies measured lucid dream frequency by using an 8-point scale ranging from "never" to "several times a week" (e.g. Schredl & Erlacher, 2004). In order to obtain units in frequency per month, the scales were recoded using the class means. Results for an online survey showed a mean lucid dream frequency of 2.81 (± 5.28) mornings per month (Erlacher & Schredl, 2005) and for a student sample a mean lucid dream frequency of 1.27 (± 2.94) mornings per month (Schredl & Erlacher, 2004) (see also Table 1).

In contrast to dream recall frequency for which stable gender differences of medium effect size have been demonstrated (Schredl & Reinhard, 2008b), large-scale surveys did not reveal any differences in lucid dream frequency between sexes (e.g. Watson, 2001). Several studies showed a considerable relationship between lucid dream frequency and dream recall frequency (e.g. Schredl & Erlacher, 2004). In addition, a significant correlation between lucid dream frequency and nightmare frequency was reported (e.g. Spadafora & Hunt, 1990). This seems plausible because a substantial portion of lucid dreamers reported that nightmares triggered lucidity within their dreams (e.g. Wolpin, Marston, Randolph, & Clothies, 1992).

It can be concluded, that about 26% of the normal population already experienced a lucid dream. Higher prevalence rates can be found in student samples. For lucid dreamers about 17% of their dreams are lucid dreams. In contrast to dream recall frequency, there is no difference between sexes for lucid dream frequency.

Table 1. Lucid dream frequency for two student samples.

	Erlacher & Schredl (n = 684)		Schredl & Erlacher (n = 439)	
Category	Frequency	Relative frequency (%)	Frequency	Relative frequency (%)
Never	113	16.5	79	18.0
Less then once a year	60	8.8	33	7.5
About once a year	44	6.4	48	10.9
About 2 to 4 times a year	113	18.0	117	26.7
About once a month	101	14.8	71	16.2
About 2 to 3 times a months	108	15.8	45	10.3
About once a week	65	9.5	35	8.0
Several times a week	70	10.2	11	2.5

2.4. Is Lucid Dreaming Related to Personality Factors?

Because lucid dreaming seems to be an extraordinary state of consciousness the question arises if this phenomenon is related to specific personality factors. The short overview presented here will focus on personality and related aspects; other factors such as vestibular balance, intelligence, and creativity are discussed extensively in Snyder and Gackenbach (1988).

Hearne (1978) hypothesized that the higher cortical activation, that could be measured during lucid dreaming compared to non-lucid REM dreams, is associated with introversion. However, this hypothesis was not supported by his own study and subsequent studies (Snyder & Gackenbach, 1988; Watson, 2001). Gackenbach, Heilman, Boyt, and LaBerge (1985) have examined the field independence construct and were able to demonstrate positive correlations to lucid dreaming frequency, although their results are mixed. These studies are based on the assumption that lucid dreamers rely on internal stimuli more often than non-lucid dreamers. One study by Blagrove and Tucker (1994) did not find a substantial relationship between field independence measured by questionnaire and lucid dreaming frequency.

Moffitt et al. (1988) suggested a correlation between meditation and lucid dreaming because the self-reflective state in meditation might stimulate lucid dreaming. Several studies supported this notion and reported a correlation between meditation frequency and lucid dream frequency (Gackenbach, 1978; Gackenbach, Cranson, & Alexander, 1986; Hunt, 1991). This is in line with the findings from Blagrove and colleagues (2000; 1994) regarding internal locus of control which these authors assume to be related to meditating. Locus of control refers to the belief in one's own control over events and their outcome. One study by Wolpin et al. (1992), however, was not able to demonstrate a positive relationship between lucid dreaming frequency and internal locus of control. In a pilot study, Prescott and Pattigrew (1995) reported a relationship between lucid dreaming frequency and a questionnaire item called "search for control over common situations in waking life". Gackenbach (1978) proposed the hypothesis that lucid dreamers are or feel in better control of their waking life. Therefore, lucid dreamers should be well-adjusted and score low on neuroticism scales. Some studies have supported this assumption, whereas the majority of studies found neuroticism or wellbeing unrelated to lucid dreaming frequency (cf. Schredl & Erlacher, 2004).

Personality dimensions such as hypnotizability and thin boundaries which can be conceptualized as subdimensions of the big five personality factor "openness to experience" were positively related to lucid dreaming frequency (cf. McCrae, 1994). This positive relationship is also given when dream recall frequency, which is also related to these dimensions (cf. Schredl, 1999), is statistically controlled for (Schredl & Erlacher, 2004).

In a more recent study by Schredl and Erlacher (2004), a random student sample was studied with respect to personality factors and lucid dream frequency. Results showed that lucid dreaming frequency was not associated with the big five personality factors (Ostendorf & Angleitner, 1994) which are neuroticism, extraversion, openness to experience, agreeableness and conscientiousness. However, substantial but small correlations were found for two openness factors ("fantasy", "ideas") and for dimensions which are associated with the openness to experience factor: Thin boundaries, Absorption and Imagination.

In summary, the studies discussed might suggest that the direct relationship between lucid dreaming frequency and personality is rather small. Thus, other variables such as meditation experience, field independence, performance of the vestibular system should be included in future models explaining interindividual differences in lucid dreaming frequency.

3. Psychophysiological Relationship During Lucid Dreams

Dreams can be considered as a kind of imagination. Both dreaming and imagination are a simulation of the real world on a higher cognitive level (Erlacher & Schredl, 2008b). This notion is supported by neuroscience studies which suggest that imagined and executed actions share the same neural substrate. Research studies on mental imagery tested this assumption on different levels: Measuring central nervous activity, monitoring autonomic response and using mental chronometry (Decety, 1996). Jeannerod (2001) integrated these findings into the theory of neural simulation of action. The simulation theory postulates that, in general, covert actions are actual actions, except for the fact that they are not executed, but share for example the same cortical areas. In the second part of this paper studies from the field of lucid dream research will be reviewed which will reveal a strong correlation between dreamed and actual actions and therefore emphasize the assumption that dreamed actions are indeed a neural simulation.

3.1. Lucid Dreaming and Central Nervous Activity

Lucid dreams offer a fascinating opportunity for studying the body-mind relationship during sleep because the dreamer can carry out pre-arranged tasks during the dream and mark their beginning and end by distinct eye movements that can be measured electrically (cf. Erlacher & Schredl, 2008b). Even the very first sleep laboratory studies about lucid dreams from Hearne (1978) and LaBerge (1980) used eye movements to validate lucid dreaming. In those studies lucid dreamers were instructed to perform eye movements in their lucid dreams (e.g. look left, right, left, right). In the corresponding EOG recording the specific eye movement patterns can be found by up and down lines. Figure 1 depicts two examples for typical lucid dream signals.

Normally, a sleeping person's body is inhibited and dreamed actions show no overt gross movements. However, electrical impulses can be measured in limb muscles which might cause small twitches (Dement & Wolpert, 1958). Several studies with lucid dreamers also demonstrated a close correlation between dreamed limb movements and EMG activities in the corresponding limb. LaBerge, Nagel, Dement, and Zarcone (1981), for example, observed that a sequence of left and right fist clenches carried out in a lucid dream resulted in a corresponding sequence of left and right forearm twitches as measured by EMG. Fenwick et al. (1984) showed that for finger and hand movements carried out in a lucid dream the EMG activity was higher than for movements which were performed with the shoulder. In proximal muscles the EMG activity can disappear at all. Several case reports by Erlacher (2007) show that the EMG activity from the forearm of a lucid dreaming person can also fade away during a series of dreamed hand movements (see Figure 1). The findings in lucid and non-lucid dreams indicate that physiological mechanisms inhibit most of the activity of the skeletal muscles that otherwise would be present due to dreamed movements.

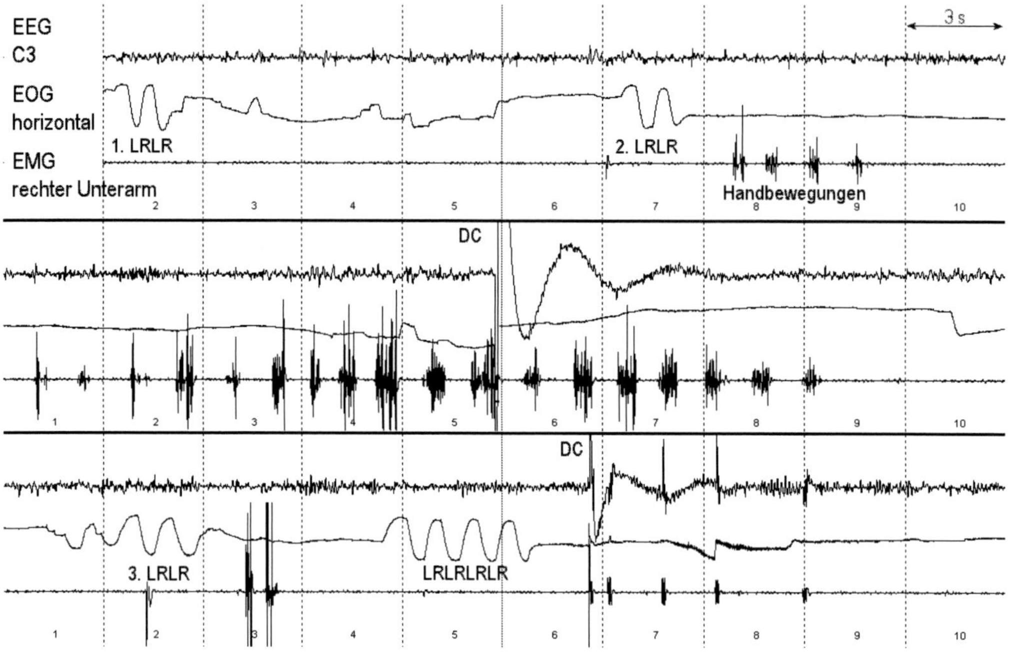

Figure 1. REM lucid dream recording. The task for the participant was to carry out hand clenches with the right hand. In his dream report the subject stated that he continuously performed hand clenches between 2. LRLR and 3. LRLR, but the EMG activity is changing throughout the recording, partially disappearing at all (from Erlacher & Schredl, 2008b)

Holzinger, LaBerge, and Levitan (2006) explored differences in EEG recordings between lucid and non-lucid dreams in REM sleep. One finding indicated a higher activation of the left parietal lobe for lucid dreams in comparison to non-lucid dreams. The authors argued that this brain area is considered to be related to semantic understanding and self-awareness and therefore reflects self awareness of the dreaming person in lucid dreams. In a study by Erlacher, Schredl, and LaBerge (2003), a single participant was instructed to carry out hand clenching either with the right or the left hand or – as a control condition – counting. Those events had to be marked by eye movements allowing for an analysis of the EEG alpha power over the motor cortex (C3, Cz and C4) for the left or right hand movements. Results showed that EEG alpha band over bilateral motor areas decreased while the lucid dreamer executed left or right hand clenching in contrast to dream counting. In general, a decrease of alpha power is assumed to indicate an activated cortical area with an increase in the excitability level of the neurones (cf. Pfurtscheller, 1992).

In a recent study, Strelen (2006) was able to evoke event related potentials during lucid dreams by using an odd-ball paradigm with an acoustic modality. During the night participants were exposed to two types of short tones (high vs. low tone). The lucid dreamers were instructed to "listen" for the high tones and signal such an event by a single left right eye movement. The analysis of three lucid dreamers who were able to accomplish this showed a P300 activation in the EEG analysis. The evoked potential (P300) can be interpreted as a conscious processing of the acoustic information during the lucid REM dreams, an EEG pattern which would also appear during wakefulness.

Voss, Holzmann, Tuin, and Hobson (2009) did a quantitative EEG study on lucid dreaming. They compared brain activation measured by EEG under three conditions: Normal dreams, lucid dreams and wakefulness. Comparison of the EEG activity between these conditions showed that the difference was located frontally, and strongest in the 40 Hz frequency band of the EEG, which was more potent in waking and lucid dreaming than it was in non-lucid dreaming. Along these results Dresler et al. (2009) conducted a pilot study using MRI techniques to study brain activation in lucid dreaming subjects. Compared to non-lucid dreaming, the regional brain activation pattern was markedly different. Lucid dreamers showed increased activation patterns not only frontally, as might have been predicted by the Voss et al. (2009) findings, but also temporal and even occipital as well.

Those recent trends in neuroscience might lead to a new line of experiments in lucid dream research with respect to consciousness in general (Hobson, 2009).

3.2. Lucid Dreaming and Physiological Changes

Dream research has shown that there is a relationship between dream content and autonomic parameters (cf. Stegie, Baust, & Engel, 1975). For example, Hobson, Goldfrank, and Snyder (1965) found a positive correlation between global dream content ratings (including ratings of emotion, physical activity, and vividness) and respiration rate as well as respiration rate variability. Baust and Engel (1971) found that large respiration amplitude correlated with intensive active participation in the dream. On the other hand, high variability of the respiration frequency was associated – in contrast to the findings from Hobson et al. – with little active participation in the dream. No correlation was found for heart rate to dream content in this study. Overall, findings in this area are inconsistent and conclusions about the relationship between dream emotions or other dream characteristics and physiological parameters cannot yet be made.

In a pilot study, LaBerge, Greenleaf, and Kedzierski (1983) showed a correspondence between subjectively experienced sexual activity during REM lucid dreaming and several autonomic parameters such as respiration rate, skin conductivity, vaginal EMG and vaginal pulse amplitude. The parameters increased significantly during experienced lucid dream orgasm, but contrary to what might be expected, heart rate increased only slightly, and the increase was not significant. Another study by LaBerge and Dement (1982) showed that lucid dreamers are able to voluntary control their respiration during lucid REM dreaming. In a study by Erlacher and Schredl (2008a) proficient lucid dreamers were instructed to carry out specific tasks (counting vs. performing squats) while lucidly dreaming. During the night heart rate and respiration rate were measured continuously. Results showed an increase of heart rate while performing squats in the lucid dream. The results with regard to respiration rate were less clear but showed the expected changes with higher respiration rates while squatting in the dream. Figure 2 shows a recording of successfully carried out squats.

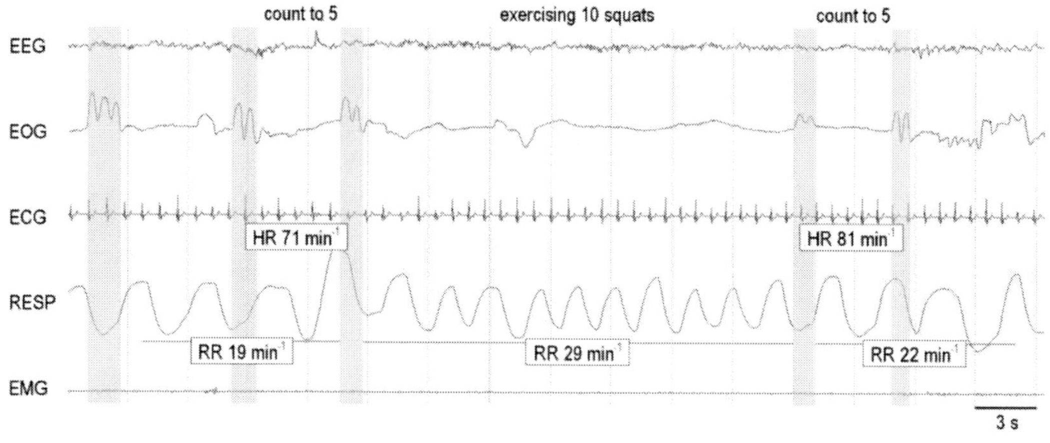

Figure 2. Recording of a lucid dream: Five clear left-right-left-right eye movement signals are shown in the EOG channel. The task for the lucid dreamer was to count from 1 to 5, perform 10 squats and finally count again from 1 to 5. As can be seen the respiration rate and heart rate increased while performing squats in the lucid dreams (from Erlacher & Schredl, 2008a).

3.3. Lucid Dreaming and Time Aspects

The relationship between subjectively estimated time in dreams and real time spent dreaming has a long history in dream research. The following dream example reported by the French sleep and dream researcher Alfred Maury (1861) raised the question whether the recalled dream is really a recollection of experiences made during sleep or is possibly generated like a flash during the process of awakening. Maury reported a long and intense dream about the French revolution which ended with the dreamer on the guillotine and the sleeper waking up with a piece of his wooden bed top having fallen on his neck. Because of the logical line of dream action, Maury hypothesized that the dream was generated backwards by the arousing stimulus.

Nowadays, it is widely accepted that the subjectively experienced time in dreams corresponds with the actual time (cf. Schredl, 2000). Dement and Kleitman (1957b) managed to demonstrate this relationship experimentally. In their study, participants were awakened in a random order either after 5 or 15 minutes of REM sleep. After awakening, participants were asked to estimate whether the elapsed sleep interval was 5 or 15 minutes. From 111 awakenings, 83 % decisions were correct. Furthermore, the elapsed time of the REM period correlated with the length of the dream report.

In a pilot study, LaBerge (1985) showed that time intervals for counting from one to ten in lucid dreams (by counting from one-thousand-and-one to one-thousand-and-ten) are close to the time intervals for counting during wakefulness. In a study by Erlacher and Schredl (2004) the time intervals for two different activities (performing squats and counting) were compared between lucid dreams and wakefulness. The results for counting confirmed LaBerge's (1985) finding that time intervals for counting were quite similar in lucid dreams and in wakefulness, but performing squats required 44.5 % more time in lucid dreams than while being awake. The authors suggested that one possible reason explaining this disproportional effect might be the different modality of the activity (cognitive vs. motor activity).

In one of our yet unpublished studies we looked at a total number of 15 lucid dreamers with respect to time spent in lucid dreams. The participant's had to count to 10, 20, and 30 or to walk 10, 20, and 30 steps during their lucid dreams. Results showed that absolute duration of counting or walking in the lucid dream takes more time than for the same tasks during wakefulness ($M = 30\%$ for Counting; $M = 50\%$ for Walking). For both conditions, however, relative timing revealed similar percentages for both conditions (highest typical error is 1.4 for Counting and 2.5 for Walking). Thus, this result supports the notion that a temporal structure for actions in lucid dreams is present, and therefore mirrors a functional equivalence between dreamed and waking activities.

Summarizing the second part of this paper, a relationship between dream content and central nervous activity measured by EEG, EOG and EMG can be demonstrated. Autonomic responses during dreams of physical activity parallel the autonomic responses to doing the actual exercise, and the timing of dreamed and actual motor actions are closely related. These findings strongly support the hypothesis that dreamed actions are indeed a neural simulation.

4. Applications of Lucid Dreaming

Based on the findings presented so far, lucid dreams can be seen as a simulation of the real world. Lucid dreamers are able to act voluntary in the simulated dream world and do what they want to do. This raises the question about practical implications of lucid dreaming. In the third part of this paper two possible applications of lucid dreaming will be presented. Other applications as creativity or problem solving are discussed in LaBerge and Rheingold (1990).

4.1. Enhancing Athletic Performance Using Lucid Dreams

Practice during lucid dreams is a novel type of mental rehearsal in which a person is using the dream state to consciously practice specific tasks without waking up (cf. Erlacher, 2007). This kind of practice can be compared to mental practice, which is well known in sport theory and sport practice (cf. Schmidt & Lee, 2005). For both types of mental rehearsal, movements are simulated with an imagined body on a cognitive level whereas the physical body remains still. In contrast to mental practice, which is performed during wakefulness, practice in lucid dreams occurs while sleeping. For mental practice several meta-analyses (cf. Driskell, Copper, & Moran, 1994) demonstrated that in general mental practice enhances performance. It seems plausible that practice in lucid dreams would have beneficial effects as well. But in contrast to the vast amount of research on mental practice, for practice in lucid dreams the empirical basis is rather small, which can be explained by the fact that lucid dreaming is a rather unknown phenomenon in the scientific sports community.

In several anecdotal reports amateur and professional athletes claimed that they used lucid dreams to improve their actual performance while being awake (e.g. Tholey, 1990). LaBerge and Rheingold (1990) reported of several amateur athletes who improved their skills during lucid dreams, e.g. a long distance runner who practiced his running technique, a tennis novice who learned his tennis serve and a woman who enhanced her skating skills. Tholey (1990), who was a German sport psychologist and a pioneer in lucid dream research, provided further examples of professional athletes (Alpine skiing, equestrian and martial arts) who used lucid dream practice on a frequent basis.

In addition to his research interests in lucid dreaming, Tholey was himself a highly skilled lucid dreamer. In an interview he reported his own experiences in lucid dream practice: “Not every single movement I do practice in my lucid dreams. In lucid dreams I rather work on my body feeling and the orientation in the three dimensional space. For example I do somersaults and feel every single muscle twitch in my dreamed body.” (Mechsner, 1994). With his lucid dream practice he improved several sport techniques in wakefulness. Further anecdotal reports from professional athletes were collected by Erlacher (2007), for example:

> Spring board diving (female, 33): „I practice complex twists and somersaults in my lucid dreams. When I do my lucid dream practice the movements feel real but if I want to I can slow down the whole sequence to focus on important details of the dive.”
>
> Sprint training (male, 38): „Then I start to push my legs to the back and to concentrate on my feet and not only to lift my knees. Immediately I feel a force in my hips which brings me forward. The hips are now much better involved in my sprint than before.“
>
> Winter sport (male, 26): „I dreamed lucidly about snowboarding, I was in a fun park and I practiced several tricks on my board. I couldn‘t do those tricks in waking life but the practice in my dreams helped me get better.“

Up to now there are very few studies that investigated possible effects of practicing in lucid dreams in a systematic way. In a qualitative study by Tholey (1981), lucid dreamers were instructed to perform different complex sport skills, like skiing or gymnastics, which the participants already knew from waking life, in their lucid dreams. Participants reported that they had no difficulties to perform those complex sport skills in their lucid dreams. This ability is a prerequisite for lucid dream practice. Furthermore, participants reported that the movements were accompanied by a pleasant feeling in the dream and that their movements improved due to the practice for both the dream state and the waking state. However, in this study, performance after dreaming was not measured.

In a quasi-experimental pre-post design study conducted by Erlacher and Schredl (Erlacher & Schredl, in press) participants were asked to practice an aiming task in their lucid dreams. For the aiming task the participants had to toss a 10-cent Euro coin into a cup. The pre test in the evening and post test in the morning consisted of 20 tosses each. Results showed a significant increase in hitting the target from pre test to post test for the group which practiced the coin-tossing task in their lucid dreams, but no increase was found for the other group. Even though confounding variables such as motivation could not be controlled for by the experimental design used, the results of this study indicate that practice in lucid dreams enhances performance in wakefulness.

4.2. Overcoming Nightmares with Lucid Dreams

As mentioned above, nightmares and lucid dreams are closely related because distressing dreams may evoke unprompted lucidity in some persons (Wolpin et al., 1992). For people who suffer from recurrent nightmares lucid dreaming seems to be a potentially useful technique to overcome nightmare because lucid dreamer can control the content of the dream and master the frightening situation (Spoormaker & Van den Bout, 2006).

In dream research several types of distressing dreams are distinguished. A nightmare is defined as an "extremely frightening dream" which awaken the sleeper (American Psychiatric Association, 2000). The waking criterion is, however, not always used for a distressing dream and some researchers suggested differing between bad dreams (without awakening) and nightmares (with awakening) with nightmares exhibiting the strongest correlations to psychopathology measures (Zadra & Donderi, 2000). Frightening dreams are often used as synonym for distressing dreams, but, studies have shown that other distressing negative emotions like anger, sadness or guilt are also prevalent negative emotions in such dreams (Zadra, Pilon, & Donderi, 2006).

In general, most persons have experienced nightmares at least once in their lifetime (Englehart & Hale, 1990; Levin, 1994). In student samples, mean nightmare frequency is about one nightmare per month (Belicki, 1992; Schredl, 2003). If adults were asked whether they suffer from nightmares, about 4% to 5% of representative Samples gave an affirmative answer (e.g. Stepansky et al., 1998).

Several cognitive-behavioral techniques are effective in reducing nightmare frequency. For example imagery rehearsal treatment (Krakow & Zadra, 2006) is a cognitive-restructuring technique in which participants are instructed to write down one specific nightmare and to change the nightmare any way they wish. Similar, in lucid dream treatment the goal of the patient is to change the nightmare but within the dream. Two components of the lucid dream treatment are necessary: First, learning to become lucid during nightmares and, second, learning to change the ongoing frightening dream in a good one. To reach the first step, participants are taught in different techniques to learn lucid dreaming (Price & Cohen, 1988). Participants then choose some feature or content of the dream that they will attempt to change when lucid, so that the distressing nightmare will be redirected to a different track with an alternative (and less fearsome) ending (Spoormaker, 2008).

So fare, beneficial effects of exposure and mastery on nightmares has been anecdotally reported. Only a few case studies have been conducted, but all have shown promising results (Spoormaker, Van den Bout, & Meijer, 2003). Spoormaker and Van den Bout (2006) conducted a randomized controlled trial and found that the nightmare frequency of lucid dream treatment group had decreased, however, lucidity was not a necessary feature in this trail. Some of the participants did experience fewer nightmares after lucid dream treatment even though they had not become lucid at all and consequently could not have lucidly altered the content of their dreams. This suggests that the sheer idea or feeling of being potentially able to control and overcome one's nightmares, might play an equally vital role for reducing nightmares (Spoormaker & Van den Bout, 2006; Zadra & Pihl, 1997).

5. Discussion and Future Directions

In this paper the author argued that dreams can be considered as a kind of simulation and that within lucid dreams this simulation can be controlled and guided by the dreamer. The first part of the paper focused on general aspects about lucid dreaming (e.g. a definition, prevalence of lucid dreaming). The second part of the paper reviewed studies conducted in the field of lucid dream research which showed that correlations between dreamed and actual actions can be found for central nervous activity, autonomic responses and time aspects. In the final part of the paper different practical applications for sports and nightmare treatment were presented. A major focus will be on motor learning in lucid dreams and the effects on waking performance.

For future lucid dream research very promising is the consistent development in research tools that can be applied, especially modern neuroimaging techniques. Comparing dream reports after awakening with brain activation patterns in this same period of sleep will shed more light on the question whether the brain regions that are necessary for carrying out actions or processing incoming information in the waking state are also active while dreaming these actions or processes. However, modern neuroimaging techniques there are not without their limitations with regard to how their results can be interpreted, the latest studies published show that those problems are solvable (cf. Dang-Vu et al., 2005). One of the most interesting lines of future research will be to study lucid dreaming by modern neuroimaging techniques. Even though it will be a challenging task for a participant to have lucid dreams in a fMRI scanner, studies in the field of motor imagery have already demonstrated that this approach offers fascinating insights into the neural structures on the cortex level (cf. Lacourse, Orr, Cramer, & Cohen, 2005).

Another point that has to be stressed is that research studies on lucid REM dreams have been proven to be very effective for investigating specific questions because lucid dreamers can be instructed to perform different tasks in the dream state and mark those events by eye movements in the EOG recording. The body of literature presented provides evidence that even complex tasks can be accomplished by lucid dreamers during their lucid dreams. Thus, besides studying lucid dreams using neuroimaging techniques another interesting perspective will be to study the interaction between the lucid dreamer and external stimuli. As shown by Strelen (2006) it is possible for participants to "hear" acoustic stimuli from the external "world" and to successfully discriminate two different tones. This is but one example of a simple way of communication between the "real world setting" (research in the sleeping lab) and the lucid dreamer in his dream world. To further extend this communication process should provide very promising research opportunities.

With respect to dream time, further research is needed to clarify the inconsistent results regarding the time aspects during dreams. Erlacher and Schredl (2004) suggested that one possible factor causing differences in time intervals might be the different modalities of the tasks (e.g., motor vs. cognitive activities) and another factor might be that the duration of the tasks was unequal. To clarify if the modality or the length of the task caused the disproportional effects, further studies should scrutinize between effects of task differences and differences in time intervals.

Last but not least, the present findings should be extended to NREM sleep. Although Antrobus (1983) has shown that these reports were on a more thought-like, abstract level and less often contained images, the amount of observed variability is considerable so that some NREM reports cannot be distinguished from REM reports. This poses the question if is it possible that visual imagery is present and eye movements are absent. Furthermore, their might be additional contribution of homeostatic and not only of circadian factors which promote the generation of NREM dreams (Wamsley & Antrobus, 2008). Unfortunately, so far very few research studies looking at mind-body interaction during NREM sleep have been conducted, thus opening up another field of research and should be pursued more extensively in the future.

From an applied perspective, in sport settings it would be interesting to collect data from professional athletes regarding their knowledge about lucid dreaming and to evaluate the possibility of practice in lucid dreams. It might be possible that a small but substantial number of athletes already use lucid dreaming to improve their performance. The representative survey on Austrian athletes (N = 1000), in which 26 % of the participants stated that they had experienced lucid dreams at least once (Stepansky et al., 1998), seems to suggest this. However, it would be interesting to see if there are sports in which it might be more promising for athletes to practice during lucid dreaming than in others. For example, athletes in sports where technique plays a vital role might benefit more than competitors in sports where conditional factors such as strength and endurance are more important. Furthermore it would be interesting to provide professional athletes induction techniques to introduce them to lucid dream practice. But it looks like it will be a very challenging task for future research, not only in sports settings but also for lucid dream research in general, to find good induction techniques to reliably induce lucid dreams at night.

6. Acknowledgments

I thank Dr. Sebastian Brückner for helpful comments and improvement of the English.

7. References

American Psychiatric Association (2000). *Diagnostic and statistical manual of mental disorders* (4th ed.). Washington: American Psychiatric Press.

Antrobus, J. (1983). REM and NREM sleep reports: Comparison of word frequencies by cognitive classes. *Psychophysiology, 20*, 562-568.

Barrett, D. (1992). Just how lucid are lucid dreams? *Dreaming, 2*, 221-228.

Belicki, K. (1992). Nightmare frequency versus nightmare distress: Relations to psychopathology and cognitive style. *Journal of Abnormal Psychology, 101*, 592-597.

Blagrove, M., & Hartnell, S. J. (2000). Lucid dreaming: Associations with internal locus of control, need for cognition and creativity. *Personality and Individual Differences, 28*, 41-47.

Blagrove, M., & Tucker, M. (1994). Individual differences in locus of control and the reporting of lucid dreaming. *Personality and Individual Differences, 16*, 981-984.

Dang-Vu, T. T., Desseilles, M., Albouy, G., Darsaud, A., Gais, S., Rauchs, G., et al. (2005). Dreaming: A neuroimaging view. *Schweizer Archiv für Neurologie und Psychatrie, 156*, 415-425.

Decety, J. (1996). Do imagined and executed actions share the same neural substrate? *Cognitive Brain Research, 3*, 87-93.

Dement, W. C., & Kleitman, N. (1957a). Cyclic variations in EEG during sleep and their relation to eye movements, body motility, and dreaming. *Electroencephalography and Clinical Neurophysiology, 9*, 673-690.

Dement, W. C., & Kleitman, N. (1957b). The relation of eye movements during sleep to dream activity: an objective method for the study of dreaming. *Journal of Experimental Psychology, 53*, 339-346.

Dement, W. C., & Wolpert, E. A. (1958). The relation of eye movements, body motility, and external stimuli to dream content. *Journal of Experimental Psychology, 55*, 543-553.

Dresler, M., Wehrle, R., Koch, S., Samann, P. G., Steiger, A., Obrig, H., et al. (2009). Dream imaging - how to read the sleeping brain. *Journal of Sleep Research, 17*, 92.

Driskell, J. E., Copper, C., & Moran, A. (1994). Does mental practice enhance performance? *Journal of Applied Psychologie, 79*, 481-492.

Englehart, R. J., & Hale, D. B. (1990). Punishment, nail-biting, and nightmares: A cross-cultural study. *Journal of Multicultural Counselling and Development, 18*, 126-132.

Erlacher, D. (2007). *Motorisches Lernen im luziden Traum: Phänomenologische und experimentelle Betrachtungen*. Saarbrücken: VDM.

Erlacher, D. (2009). Recall of a specific word list in lucid dreams: An explorative online study. *International Journal of Dream Research, 2*, 37-40.

Erlacher, D., & Schredl, M. (2004). Time required for motor activity in lucid dreams. *Perceptual and Motor Skills, 99*, 1239-1242.

Erlacher, D., & Schredl, M. (2005). Online-Experiment: Erinnerung im luziden Traum. *Unveröffentlichte Daten: Universität Heidelberg*.

Erlacher, D., & Schredl, M. (2008a). Cardiovascular responses to dreamed physical exercise during REM lucid dreaming. *Dreaming, 18*, 112-121.

Erlacher, D., & Schredl, M. (2008b). Do REM (lucid) dreamed and executed actions share the same neural substrate? *International Journal of Dream Research, 1*, 7-13.

Erlacher, D., & Schredl, M. (in press). Practicing a motor task in a lucid dream enhances subsequent performance: A pilot study. *The Sport Psychologist*.

Erlacher, D., Schredl, M., & LaBerge, S. (2003). Motor area activation during dreamed hand clenching: A pilot study on EEG alpha band. *Sleep and Hypnosis, 5*, 182-187.

Erlacher, D., Schredl, M., Watanabe, T., Yamana, J., & Ganzert, F. (2008). The incidence of lucid dreaming within a Japanese university student sample. *International Journal of Dream Research, 1*, 39-43.

Fenwick, P., Schatzmann, M., Worsley, A., Adams, J., Stone, S., & Backer, A. (1984). Lucid dreaming: Correspondence between dreamed and actual events in one subject during REM sleep. *Biological Psychology, 18*, 243-252.

Gackenbach, J. (1978). *A personality and cognitive style analysis of lucid dreaming.* University of Richmond.

Gackenbach, J., Cranson, R., & Alexander, C. (1986). Lucid dreaming, witnessing, and the transcendental meditation: A developmental relationship. *Lucidity Letter, 5*, 34-41.

Gackenbach, J., Heilman, N., Boyt, S., & LaBerge, S. (1985). The relationship between field independence and lucid dreaming ability. *Journal of Mental Imagery, 9*, 9-20.

Gillespie, G. (1984). Can we distinguish between lucid dreams and dreaming awareness dreams? *Lucidity Letter, 3*, 9-11.

Hearne, K. M. (1978). *Lucid dreams: an electrophysiological and psychological study.* University of Liverpool, Liverpool.

Hobson, A. J. (2009). The neurobiology of consciousness: Lucid dreaming wakes up. *International Journal of Dream Research, 2*, 41-44.

Hobson, J. A., Goldfrank, F., & Snyder, F. (1965). Respiration and mental activity in sleep. *Journal of psychiatric research, 3*, 79-90.

Hobson, J. A., & Pace-Schott, E. F. (2002). The cognitive neuroscience of sleep: Neuronal systems, consciousness and learning. *Nature Reviews Neuroscience, 3*, 679-693.

Hobson, J. A., Pace-Schott, E. F., & Stickgold, R. (2000). Dreaming and the brain: Toward a cognitive neuroscience of conscious states. *Behavioral and Brain Sciences, 23*, 793-842.

Holzinger, B., LaBerge, S., & Levitan, L. (2006). Psychophysiological correlates of lucid dreaming. *Dreaming, 16*, 88-95.

Hunt, H. T. (1991). Lucid dreaming as a meditative state: Some evidence from long-term meditators in relation to the cognitive-psychological bases of transpersonal phenomena. In J. Gackenbach, & A. A. Sheikh (Eds.), Dream images: A call to mental arms (pp. 265-285). Amityville, New York: Baywood.

Jeannerod, M. (2001). Neural simulation of action: A unifying mechanism for motor cognition. *Neuroimage, 14*, 103-109.

Krakow, B., & Zadra, A. (2006). Clinical Management of Chronic Nightmares: Imagery Rehearsal Therapy. *Behavioral Sleep Medicine, 4*, 45-70.

LaBerge, S. (1980). *Lucid dreaming: An exploratory study of consciousness during sleep.* Stanford University, Palo Alto, CA.

LaBerge, S. (1985). *Lucid dreaming. The power of being awake and aware in your dreams.* Los Angeles: Tarcher.

LaBerge, S., & Dement, W. C. (1982). Lateralization of alpha activity for dreamed singing and counting during REM sleep. *Psychophysiology, 19*, 331-332.

LaBerge, S., Greenleaf, W., & Kedzierski, B. (1983). Physiological responses to dreamed sexual activity during REM sleep. *Psychophysiology, 19*, 454-455.

LaBerge, S., Nagel, L. E., Dement, W. C., & Zarcone, V. P. (1981). Lucid dreaming verified by volitional communication during REM sleep. *Perceptual and Motor Skills, 52*, 727-732.

LaBerge, S., & Rheingold, H. (1990). *Exploring the world of lucid dreams.* New York: Ballantine.

Lacourse, M. G., Orr, E. L. R., Cramer, S. C., & Cohen, M. J. (2005). Brain activation during execution and motor imagery of novel and skilled sequential hand movements. *Neuroimage, 27*, 505-519.

Levin, R. (1994). Sleep and dream characteristics of frequent nightmare subjects in a universitary population. *Dreaming, 4*, 127-137.

Maury, A. (1861). *Le sommeil et les reves.* Paris: Didier.

McCrae, R. R. (1994). Openness to experience: Expanding the boundaries of factor V. *European Journal of Personality, 8*, 251-272.

Mechsner, F. (1994). Geschichten aus der Nacht. *Geo*, 12-30.

Moffitt, A., Hoffmann, R., Mullington, J., Purcell, S., Pigeau, R., & Wells, R. (1988). Dream psychology: Operating in the dark. In J. Gackenbach, & S. LaBerge (Eds.), Conscious Mind, Sleeping Brain (pp. 429-439). New York: Plenum.

Ostendorf, F., & Angleitner, A. (1994). A comparison of different instruments proposed to measure the Big Five. *European Review of Applied Psychology, 44*, 45-53.

Pfurtscheller, G. (1992). Event-related synchronization (ERS): an electrophysiological correlate of cortical areas at rest. *Electroencephalography and Clinical Neurophysiology, 83*, 62-69.

Prescott, J. A., & Pettigrew, C. G. (1995). Lucid dreaming and control in waking life. *Perceptual and Motor Skills, 81*, 658.

Price, R. F., & Cohen, D. B. (1988). Lucid dream induction. An empirical evaluation. In J. Gackenbach, & S. LaBerge (Eds.), Conscious Mind, Sleeping Brain (pp. 105-134). New York: Plenum.

Rechtschaffen, A., & Kales, A. (1968). *A manual of standarized terminology, techniques and scoring system for sleep stages of human subjects*. Washington: U. S. Public Health Service.

Roffwarg, H. P., Dement, W. C., Muzio, J. N., & Fischer, C. (1962). Dream imagery: relationship to rapid eye movements of sleep. *Archives of general psychiatry, 7*, 235-258.

Schmidt, R. A., & Lee, T. D. (2005). *Motor Control and Learning. A Behavioral Emphasis* (4. ed.). Champaign: Human Kinetics.

Schredl, M. (1999). *Die nächtliche Traumwelt: Eine Einführung in die psychologische Traumforschung*. Stuttgart: Kohlhammer.

Schredl, M. (2000). Body-mind interaction: Dream content and REM sleep physiology. *North American Journal of Psychology, 2*, 59-70.

Schredl, M. (2003). Effects of state and trait factors on nightmare frequency. *European Archives of Psychiatry and Clinical Neuroscience, 253*, 241-247.

Schredl, M., & Erlacher, D. (2003). The problem of dream content analysis validity as shown by a bizarreness scale. *Sleep and Hypnosis, 5*, 129-135.

Schredl, M., & Erlacher, D. (2004). Lucid dreaming frequency and personality. *Personality and Individual Differences, 37*, 1463-1473.

Schredl, M., & Hofmann, F. (2003). Continuity between waking activities and dream activities. *Consciousness and Cognition, 12*, 298-308.

Schredl, M., & Reinhard, I. (2008a). Dream recall, dream length, and sleep duration: State or trait factor. *Perceptual and Motor Skills, 106*, 633636.

Schredl, M., & Reinhard, I. (2008b). Gender differences in dream recall: A meta-analysis. *Journal of Sleep Research, 17*, 125-131.

Schredl, M., & Wittmann, L. (2005). Dreaming: A psychological view. *Schweizer Archiv für Neurologie und Psychatrie, 156*, 484-492.

Snyder, T. J., & Gackenbach, J. (1988). Individual differences associated with lucid dreaming. In J. Gackenbach, & S. LaBerge (Eds.), Conscious Mind, Sleeping Brain (pp. 221-259). New York: Plenum.

Spadafora, A., & Hunt, H. T. (1990). The multiplicity of dreams: Cognitive-affective correlates of lucid, archetypal and nightmare dreaming. *Perceptual and Motor Skills, 71*, 627-644.

Spoormaker, V. I. (2008). A cognitive model of recurrent nightmares. *International Journal of Dream Research, 1*, 15-22.

Spoormaker, V. I., & Van den Bout, J. (2006). Lucid dreaming treatment for nightmares: A pilot study. *Psychotherapy and Psychosomatics, 75*, 389-394.

Spoormaker, V. I., Van den Bout, J., & Meijer, E. J. G. (2003). Lucid dreaming treatment for nightmares: A series of cases. *Dreaming, 13*, 181-186.

Stegie, R., Baust, W., & Engel, R. R. (1975). Psychophysiological correlates in dreams. In W. Koella (Ed.), Sleep 1974 (pp. 409-412). Basel: Karger.

Stepansky, R., Holzinger, B., Schmeiser-Rieder, A., Saletu, B., Kunze, M., & Zeitlhofer, J. (1998). Austrian's dream behavior: Results of a representative population survey. *Dreaming, 8*, 23-31.

Strelen, J. (2006). *Akustisch evozierte Potentiale bei luziden Träumen*. University of Mainz: Unpublished doctoral thesis.

Tart, C. T. (1984). Terminology in lucid dream research. *Lucidity Letter, 3*, 4-6.

Tholey, P. (1981). Empirische Untersuchungen ueber Klarträume. *Gestalt Theory, 3*, 21-62.

Tholey, P. (1988). Overview of the German research in the field of lucid dreaming. *Lucidity Letter, 7*, 26-29.

Tholey, P. (1990). Applications of lucid dreaming in sports. *Lucidity Letter, 9*, 6-17.

Voss, U., Holzmann, R., Tuin, I., & Hobson, A. J. (2009). Lucid dreaming: A state of consciousness with features of both waking and non-lucid dreaming. *Sleep, 32*, 1191-1200.

Wamsley, E., & Antrobus, J. S. (2008). Homeostatic and circadian influences on dreaming: NREM mentation during a short daytime nap. *International Journal of Dream Research, 1*, 27-33.

Watson, D. (2001). Dissociations of the night: individual differences in sleep-related experiences and their relation to dissociation and schizotypy. *Journal of Abnormal Psychology, 110*, 526-535.

Wolpin, M., Marston, A., Randolph, C., & Clothies, A. (1992). Individual differences correlates of reported lucid dreaming frequency and control. *Journal of Mental Imagery, 16*, 231-236.

Zadra, A., & Donderi, D. C. (2000). Nightmares and bad dreams: Their prevalence and relationship to well-being. *Journal of Abnormal Psychology, 109*, 273-281.

Zadra, A., Pilon, M., & Donderi, D. C. (2006). Variety and intensity of emotions in nightmares and bad dreams. *Journal of Nervous and Mental Disease, 194*, 249-254.

Zadra, A. L., Donderi, D. C., & Pihl, R. O. (1992). Efficacy of lucid dream induction for lucid and non-lucid dreamers. *Dreaming, 2*, 85-97.

Zadra, A. L., & Pihl, R. O. (1997). Lucid dreaming as a treatment for recurrent nightmares. *Psychotherapy and Psychosomatics, 66*, 50-55.

INDEX

A

B

C

D

E

F

G

H

I

J

K

L

M

N

O

P

Q

R

S

T